PSYCHIATRIC ASPECTS OF CRIMINAL BEHAVIOR

Collected Papers of Eugene Revitch

PSYCHIATRIC ASPECTS OF CRIMINAL BEHAVIOR

Collected Papers of Eugene Revitch

Edited by

LOUIS B. SCHLESINGER, PH.D.

Professor of Forensic Psychology
John Jay College of Criminal Justice
City University of New York

CHARLES C THOMAS • PUBLISHER, LTD
Springfield • Illinois • U.S.A.

Published and Distributed Throughout the World by

CHARLES C THOMAS • PUBLISHER, LTD.
2600 South First Street
Springfield, Illinois 62704

ISBN 978-0-398-09145-3 (paper)
ISBN 978-0-398-09146-0 (ebook)

With THOMAS BOOKS *careful attention is given to all details of manufacturing and design. It is the Publisher's desire to present books that are satisfactory as to their physical qualities and artistic possibilities and appropriate for their particular use.* THOMAS BOOKS *will be true to those laws of quality that assure a good name and good will.*

Printed in the United States of America
TO-C-1

Library of Congress Cataloging-in-Publication Data

Names: Revitch, Eugene, 1909-1996, author. | Schlesinger, Louis B., editor.
Title: Psychiatric aspects of criminal behavior : collected papers of Eugene Revitch / edited by Louis B. Schlesinger.
Description: Springfield, Illinois : Charles C. Thomas, Publisher, LTD., [2017] | Includes bibliographical references.
Identifiers: LCCN 2016044950 (print) | LCCN 2016045384 (ebook) | ISBN 9780398091453 (paper) | ISBN 9780398091460 (ebook)
Subjects: | MESH: Criminal Behavior | Sex Offenses--psychology | Epilepsy--psychology | Paranoid Disorders--psychology | Physician-Patient Relations | Collected Works | Case Reports
Classification: LCC HV6080 (print) | LCC HV6080 (ebook) | NLM WM 605 | DDC 364.3--dc23
LC record available at https://lccn.loc.gov/2016044950

INTRODUCTION

We often hear that scientific knowledge gained today–methods currently in use as well as recent research–is outdated after about 10 years. This is an overstatement and simply incorrect. Although many of Doctor Revitch's papers were published 50 years ago, they are as relevant today as when they first appeared. I edited this book because I did not want these seminal papers to become lost in the archives, to be only referenced in term papers or literature reviews. When I trained, I read and reread these articles many times, always learning something new. These works were so important to me in learning about various types of criminal behavior that I simply could not allow them to become abandoned and forgotten. It would serve students well including established professionals, to obtain a fundamental understanding of some of the most complex forms of human behavior by studying these important papers which astutely describe various clinical conditions.

I met Doctor Revitch on the first day of my clinical internship in 1973 at the New Jersey State Diagnostic Center. He was the person at the Center in charge of training, and all psychiatry residents and clinical psychology interns attended his bi-weekly staff meetings. His desk was in the center of the office, in front of a large window, and along the remaining three walls were chairs filled with staffers and trainees. While leading a discussion of the case that was presented, Doctor Revitch was also dictating a report, answering a phone call about an "interesting case," referencing Dostoyevsky's Raskolnikov and, at the same time, interpreting an EEG. And throughout, he frequently commented on the disintegration of Western society! To say that Doctor Revitch was a multitasker is an understatement. He finally left the meeting abruptly in order to handle a consultation at JFK Hospital about a quarter-mile away, and then to attend to his private patients in the afternoon. Most of the trainees were left sitting there overwhelmed, but I was very impressed.

Notwithstanding the disorganization, I immediately observed a brilliant psychiatrist who explained cases in a substantive way rather than with psychobabble. Up to this point in my training, I had many supervisors who seemed, to me, to really not understand the psychopathology and psychodynamics of a case, but rather just made things up that sounded good. At that point in my training, I did not know what was correct, but I believed that much of what I had heard was incorrect. I knew if I could tolerate Doctor Revitch's authoritarian style, dogmatic approach, and blunt criticism, I could learn a great deal. I asked him whether I could sit in on his evaluations and I was able to also attend his courtroom testimony in a murder trial. In addition, I also observed several sodium amytal interviews. On one occasion, he demonstrated the "cheap" needles that were being used, by bending one while it was in the defendant's vein–just another indication of the weakening standards and harmful effects of state government bureaucracy!

Doctor Revitch was my teacher and mentor, and later we became colleagues and friends. We wrote several books together in the 1980s–*Psychopathology of Homicide* (1981), *Sexual Dynamics of Anti-Social Behavior* (1983), and *Sex Murder and Sex Aggression* (1989)–as well as several book chapters, and we worked together on many interesting cases. At the end of his career, as he stopped taking on forensic cases, I was simultaneously beginning to establish my own career and getting many fascinating referrals. I spoke to Doctor Revitch weekly until the end of his life to discuss cases–forensic and clinical cases as well–and I learned something from every conversation.

Doctor Revitch has been a part of my professional career from day one. As I now enter the latter stages of my own career, I am still immersed in his work. His ideas have been with me for over forty years, and his papers are still in organized piles on my bookshelf.

In academia, a *Festschrift* is a book honoring a respected person, and is presented to him or her during the honoree's lifetime. A comparable book, presented posthumously, is a *Gedenkschrift*–a memorial publication. This edited *Gedenkschrift* of Doctor Revitch's collected papers is a modest attempt to honor a truly distinguished man.

Louis B. Schlesinger, Ph.D.
Maplewood, N.J.
August, 2016

EUGENE REVITCH, M.D.
(1909-1996)

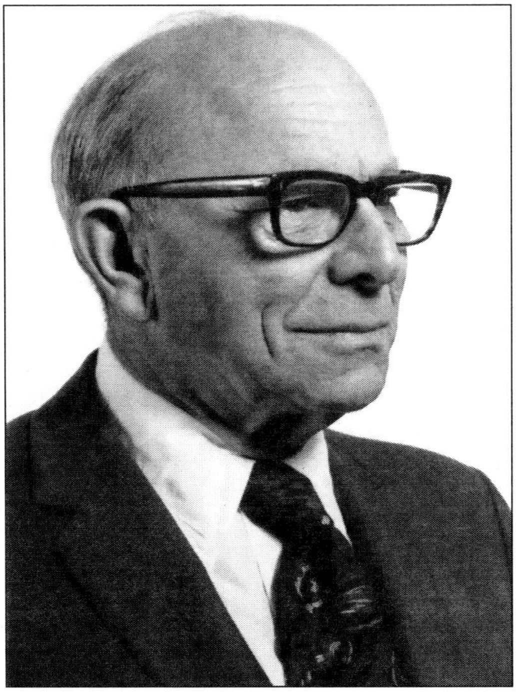

Eugene Revitch was born in Dubulti, Latvia, in 1909. At that time, Nicholas II was still the czar of Russia, Franz Joseph was the emperor of the Austro-Hungarian state, and most European countries, except for France and Switzerland, were still kingdoms and not republics. When Doctor Revitch was about five years old, the Russians–who controlled Latvia at that time–thought his family members were German spies, or would support Germany in a war against Russia, and the family was forced to leave the country. In 1920, they were all able to return to Latvia.

Doctor Revitch was raised in a middle-class family which included his sister and two brothers. His father was self-educated and initially worked as a tutor for wealthy children; he later became a businessman and, with a partner, began an import-export textile business, which eventually included a small factory and a retail store. His mother was a homemaker.

Doctor Revitch's interest in medicine began at an early age. It seems his father was diagnosed as having Meniere's disease, an illness of the inner ear that affected his balance. From his experience observing the doctors evaluate his father's condition and arrive at a diagnosis, as well as an operation he had on his hand a year previously, Doctor Revitch's initial interest in zoology and the wildlife on the African continent changed to an interest in medicine. Doctor Revitch graduated from the gymnasium (the United States equivalent of high school with an academic emphasis) in 1928, at 19 years of age. He decided to study medicine in France because he viewed France as the center of Europe and as more connected with the rest of the world than some other countries with medical schools.

He first attended the University of Montpellier, located in an ancient university town in southern France. The medical school was founded at the end of the twelfth century and was the second medical school established in Europe. At that time, medical school was five years preceded by one year of premedical studies which consisted of physics, chemistry and natural sciences (zoology and botany). College was not a prerequisite for the study of medicine (or law) in Europe, as it was in the United States. After completing his premedical studies, Doctor Revitch attended his first year of medical school at Montpellier, but decided to transfer to the University of Paris for the rest of his medical training. He believed that the cosmopolitan aspect of the French capital, as well as a degree from a school in Paris, would have greater significance abroad. Also, the fact that his friend had transferred to the University of Paris law school, probably played a role in this decision as well.

Doctor Revitch had his neurology training with the renowned George C. Guillain. Professor Guillain–most noted for the Guillain-Barre syndrome–occupied the same chair, in the same hospital, as did Jean-Martin Charcot in the 1800s. Every Tuesday students crowded into the room where Charcot presented his patients. Among his students was Sigmund Freud who studied with Charcot on a fellowship in 1885. During 1934 to 1935, Doctor Revitch worked on his doctoral thesis, a requirement of European medical schools at that time. He initially wanted to study childhood tuberculosis, but switched his topic to the study of the effect of war gases, which he thought might be more relevant to the future. He completed his thesis and his examinations, and graduated with a degree in medicine in 1935.

On his trip home from Paris to Latvia, Doctor Revitch read an article in a medical journal about a newly introduced brain-wave test, the electroencephalogram. It fascinated him, and it reinforced his intense interest in neurology. Once back in Latvia, he was drafted into the Latvian army. He was a private in the ski-and-bicycle infantry unit, serving on the Russian border. Following discharge, he realized that there was no future for him in Europe, and he decided to emigrate to the United States in 1938, where he joined relatives who had already settled in Philadelphia.

Once Doctor Revitch arrived in the United States, he had difficulty obtaining an internship, which is a requirement to become a licensed physician. At that time, organized medicine kept tight control on the number of physicians allowed to practice, and the medical establishment was especially questioning of foreign medical graduates. Ostensibly, this skepticism was for quality-control purposes, but it was really primarily for economic reasons–to keep the supply of physicians low so that the demand for services would be high. Before securing an internship, Doctor Revitch worked at a few jobs, including assisting in a tuberculosis research project at the Phipps Institute in Philadelphia. Finally, after mailing about two hundred letters to various hospitals in the United States, he got an internship in 1939 at St. Peter's General Hospital in New Brunswick, New Jersey. This internship lasted about two and a half years; during which he not only learned a great deal about general medicine, but he also realized how little attending physicians knew about, or understood, psychiatric disorders.

Following his internship, Doctor Revitch took a residency in psychiatry at the Institute of Pennsylvania Hospital in Philadelphia. He was always an astute observer of people, and he noticed that many of his fellow residents, as well as practicing psychiatrists, seemed to be enamored with psychoanalysis which, at that time, was the Cadillac of psychiatric practice, especially private practice. However, he found that many of his colleagues had only a superficial connection to psychoanalysis, as they just tried to imitate a stereotypical psychoanalytic role such as remaining silent, being inactive, and not giving any advice or support to patients. He concluded that psychodynamic concepts were useful, but that the inactive approach was unhelpful–and sometimes harmful–to many patients. Instead of pursuing psychoanalysis, he became increasingly interested in neuropsychiatry and forensic psychiatry.

During this time, Doctor Revitch was becoming extremely anxious about the war in Europe, and he decided to join the U. S. Army–his second stint in military service. He had a number of assignments in the military, but the one that seemed to be most significant–and which he spoke about even towards the end of his life–was his time as an army psychiatrist at the disciplinary barracks in Missoula, Montana. Here, he was able to evaluate murderers, rapists, and other offenders. His observation at that time, which proved to be absolutely correct years later, was that those individuals who committed nonhomicidal offenses were more unstable and disturbed than the majority of the murderers. In fact, many of the most dangerous individuals were polite and seemed normal, on the surface, but they engaged in some very disturbed and violent acts.

Following military service, Doctor Revitch took a job at the Lyons V.A. Hospital in New Jersey, as many military physicians were recruited by the Veteran's Administration following World War II. While a staff psychiatrist at Lyons, he was able to avail himself of the many training opportunities at the V.A. and he participated in a good deal of the training with the neurology residents. He attended neurology lectures at the Neurological Institute in New York, and was in residence for about five months at the National Veteran's Epilepsy Center in Massachusetts, serving as a footing for his intense interest in epileptoid violence and psychiatric aspects of epilepsy.

In 1952, Doctor Revitch joined staff of the newly established New Jersey State Diagnostic Center, in Menlo Park, which was created to evaluate sex offenders as well as to assess all sorts of criminal and complex marital cases. Doctor Revitch used his experience at the disciplinary barracks as a foundation for his work at the Diagnostic Center. While at the Center, he perfected the technique of sodium amytal interviews and became interested in the prison system, and the interface between psychiatry and law. He spent hours working on many interesting cases. Doctor Revitch remarked that, over the years, he developed a low opinion of lawyers, but a high opinion of detectives. He found that detectives were interested in the nature of the crimes they investigated, and his discussions with detectives were a productive exchange of opinions and experiences. In contrast, Doctor Revitch found that his contacts with attorneys almost always resulted in some type of legalistic and semantic argument over topics such as insanity and competency, which just frustrated him.

After about 23 years of service at the Diagnostic Center he left, as the institution closed, and he went into full-time private practice for the remainder of his career. Over the years, in addition to his general psychiatric and neuropsychiatric practice, he was involved in many forensic cases that included courtroom testimony. A retired criminal court judge told me several years after Doctor Revitch's death that he found him an easy witness to cross-examine, because "he was so honest."

Doctor Revitch was also a clinical professor of psychiatry at the Robert Wood Johnson, Medical School in Piscataway and, in 1967, he founded and became the director of the psychiatry department at the John F. Kennedy Medical Center in Edison. He was also a consultant in electroencephalography and psychiatry at Lyons V.A. Hospital, and a consultant at Muhlenberg Hospital as well.

Doctor Revitch made a substantial impact not only on the lives of his many students and patients, but also on the field of neuropsychiatry and forensic psychiatry. He led a fascinating life. He spoke seven languages and was a true intellectual. All those who knew Doctor Revitch, even casually or briefly, found him to be an unforgettable character.

Sadly, during World War II, Doctor Revitch lost all his immediate family, except for his sister. His parents were executed in Latvia in 1941, and his younger brothers died fighting the Germans as members of the Red Army. His sister survived the Bergen-Belsen concentration camp and was able to come to the United States following the war. Notwithstanding these tragic events, Doctor Revitch was never bitter nor did he ever describe these losses in an angry, astringent, or resentful way. Doctor Revitch retired in 1987 because of severe visual problems and the development of Alzheimer's disease. He died in 1996 after a lifetime of enormous achievement and service.

CONTENTS

SECTION III. PSYCHIATRIC ASPECTS OF EPILEPSY AND EPILEPTOID VIOLENCE

PSYCHIATRIC ASPECTS OF CRIMINAL BEHAVIOR

Collected Papers of Eugene Revitch

Section I

SEX MURDER AND SEX AGGRESSION

INTRODUCTION

When Eugene Revitch published *Sex Murder and Sex Aggression* in 1957, little scientific literature existed on the topic, except perhaps for Richard von Krafft-Ebing's (1886) *Psychopathia Sexualis* and Magnus Hirschfeld's (1944) *Sexual Anomalies and Perversions.* Some early work on sex offenders (who did not commit homicide) was available, and Doctor Revitch's colleagues at the New Jersey Diagnostic Center–Albert Ellis and Ralph Brancale–had just published their landmark text (1956), *The Psychology of Sex Offenders.* Sex murder and sex aggression constituted essentially new ground from a psychiatric or psychological perspective, and the general public had hardly any interest in the topic. This situation is dramatically different today, as the media are saturated with both fictional stories and true-crime documentaries about all aspects of sexual and serial sexual murderers.

Doctor Revitch's (1957) paper is truly a seminal work, particularly his classification of the aggressive expression of sexual instincts into four groups: murder as a prerequisite for sexual satisfaction; murder not as a prerequisite for sexual satisfaction but due to frustration, anger, or fear during attempted intercourse or rape; aggressive sexual needs expressed in knifing, slugging, or choking with or without ejaculation; and aggressive sexual needs expressed only in fantasy life. In this paper, Doctor Revitch described the compulsive-repetitive nature of some sexual murders, and he also stated his belief that the prognosis in such cases is difficult to make. He argued for additional clinical research, for the courts to refer such cases for evaluation, and for sexually aggressive acts by children to serve as red flags.

Extreme Manifestations of Sexual Aggression, published in 1965, described the sexual nature of some unprovoked assaults on and murders of women by men. In this paper, Doctor Revitch first cited the work of Frederick Wertham (1949) regarding murders associated with a tension release that Wertham had described in his earlier work (1937) under the name *catathymic crisis*. Doctor Revitch again asked the judiciary to be alert and aware of red flags that signaled some individuals' potential to commit sexually aggressive acts.

Also, in 1965 Doctor Revitch wrote "Sex Murder and the Potential Sex Murderer," in which he reported his empirical study of 43 men (whom he personally examined) who carried out sexual attacks on women, including murder. The author described the psychodynamics in such cases, as well as disposition and management recommendations, and he reviewed cases involving evisceration, severe mutilation, and cannibalism. He concluded that fetishism of female underwear, solo breaking-and-entering under bizarre circumstances, sadistic fantasies, minor assaults on women, and mutilation of animals are important prognostic signs. He discussed problems connected with the sentencing of such dangerous offenders and the need to establish specialized diagnostic facilities to handle these cases.

Doctor Revitch's keynote address to the Association of Corrective and Social Psychiatrists was published as a paper in 1980 under the title "Gynocide and Unprovoked Attacks on Women." Here, the author discussed the phenomenology, diagnosis, and classification of compulsive, sexually motivated acts, including murder, and provided numerous illustrative cases. He also expanded on the concept of catathymic homicides and assaults, based on the earlier (1937) work of Wertham. Again, Doctor Revitch reviewed the warning signs of potential sex murderers and advised that the prognostic significance of such signs and characteristics, especially when seen in combination, be used to alert authorities about potential gynocidal offenders. In this paper, Doctor Revitch also touched on a possible neurobiological underpinning of sexual violence, based on the work of Paul D. MacLean (1962)–specifically, anatomical structures in the limbic system connecting sex with aggression.

Sexual burglaries are a phenomenon first described and studied by Doctor Revitch. The last two chapters in Section I are two of his papers on this topic. In his 1978 paper, Doctor Revitch discussed those relatively rare burglaries that are not committed for any type of gain, but are sexually motivated. He discussed voyeuristic impulses in breaking-and- entering, when offenders have an urge to look around and open and inspect drawers, with the fantasy of seeing a naked woman or while entertaining various other voyeuristic fantasies. Doctor Revitch drew clear distinction between gain-oriented repetitive burglaries and those that are sexually motivated. And he offered an important investigative recommendation–in cases of bizarre sexual murders of women, burglars with a history of minor attacks on women should be considered as the perpetrator, rather than typical sex offenders, who are mostly pedophiles, who generally do not carry out sex murders.

In the last chapter of this section, Doctor Revitch expanded on his view of burglaries with sexual dynamics. He reported seven cases and discussed all of them in considerable depth. He cited Freud's (1919) concept of the repetition compulsion as a possible explanation for the dynamics of some of these compulsively driven offenses. Doctor Revitch also reported the value of interviewing offenders under the influence of intravenously injected sodium amytal (a method which he perfected) in order to fully understand the dynamics of such cases. Doctor Revitch concluded that purely legal procedures will not protect the public or even help pathological perpetrators with rehabilitation if that is possible.

REFERENCES

Ellis, A., & Brancale, R. (1956). *The psychology of sex offenders.* Springfield, IL: Charles C Thomas.

Freud, S. (1919). Beyond the pleasure principle. *Collected papers, Vol. xviii.* London: Hogarth Press.

Hirschfeld, M. (1944). *Sexual anomalies and perversions.* London: Francis Aldor Publishers.

Krafft-Ebing, R. von (1886). *Psychopathia Sexualis.* Philadelphia: F. A. Davis.

MacLean, P. P. (1962). New finding relevant to the evolution of the psycho-sexual functions of the brain. *Journal of Nervous and Mental Disease, 135*: 289-301.

Wertham, F. (1937). The catathymic crisis: A clinical entity. *Archives of Neurology and psychiatry, 37*:974-977.

Wertham, F. (1949). *The show of violence.* New York: Doubleday.

Chapter 1

SEX MURDER AND SEX AGGRESSION

Two recent sex murders in New Jersey aroused public and official concern about our ability to prognosticate sexual violence. Although aggressive sexual acts make the headlines, initial studies by Brancale[1] and others[2,3] confirm what seems to be the impression of psychiatrists working in the field: that the majority of sex offenders are innocuous, inadequate, passive, individuals committing minor offenses. Exhibitionism, dissemination of obscene material, noncoital relations with immature boys and girls and statutory rape are the most frequent sex offenders referred by the courts to the New Jersey State Diagnostic Center. Although Karpman[4] quotes Hartwell by saying that many sex murders of children are committed by pedophiles, Brancale[5] in his extensive experience saw only one such case. In my own experience, the only case was that of a fifteen-year-old boy murdering a six-year-old girl during or after rape. As a matter of fact, true pedophiles belong to the most passive group of sex offenders and their acts consist of noncoital relationships with children such as kissing, touching, fingering genitals of little girls and the like. Furthermore, Rogers and Weiss[6] found that in many instances, "victims" are such in the legal sense only, since due to their own emotional needs, they induce the emotionally inadequate pedophiles into sexual play. This study confirms my personal clinical impression. Davidson[7] points out that aggressive sexuality may manifest itself in symbolic acts of nonsexual nature such as pyromania, or sexual motives may be elicited in general crimes such as murder. It is not too uncommon to encounter dangerous sexual compulsions under the guise of common crimes.

Source: Revitch, E. (1957). Sex Murder and Sex Aggression. *Journal of the Medical Society of New Jersey*, *11*:519-523.

1. For the sake of this study, the aggressive expressions of the sexual instinct will be divided into four groups:
2. Murder is the prerequisite of sexual satisfaction.
3. Murder is not a prerequisite for sexual satisfaction but is due to frustration, anger or fear during an attempt at intercourse or rape.
4. The aggressive sexual needs are expressed in knifing, slugging or choking, with or without ejaculation during the act.
4. The aggressive sexual needs are expressed in phantasy life only.

These four categories are not fixed. History is replete with cases in which unprovoked assaults, beatings or chokings eventually transform into repetitive murders of Group 1. In some instances, these murders are preceded by a long history of disorganized behavior. Murders in Group 1 connected with mutilation of the body and even anthropophagy (eating of human flesh) have been reported in psychiatric literature by authors of the last century.[8] One of the outstanding cases is that of Vincent Verzeni, examined by Lombroso and quoted by Krafft-Ebing.[8] Verzeni was arrested in 1872 at the age of 23 years for an attempt to strangle his nurse while she was lying sick in bed, and also for similar attempts on three other women. After his arrest, it was discovered that he had killed a 14-year old girl, mutilated her body, tore out her intestines and genitals, bit off a piece of flesh from the right calf and sucked the blood from the wound. He had strangled a twenty-eight-year-old woman and ripped out her intestines. He had dragged his 19-year-old cousin into the fields and tried to choke her. He took a portion of flesh from one of his victim's home to roast and eat, but later he changed his mind and hid it, since he was afraid his mother might discover his behavior. After his arrest, Verzeni explained that he had an "unspeakable delight" in strangling women and that during the act he experienced erection and ejaculation.

That repetitive killing of victims may be preceded by abnormal aggressive behavior is well illustrated in the case of Heirens,[9] a 17-year-old student who killed two women and then kidnapped a six-year-old girl and dismembered her body. At the age of nine, Heirens began stealing female undergarments. Later on he committed burglaries, originally not to obtain female undergarments, and later because of a sexual thrill accompanied with ejaculation while he entered a home through the window.[9] He struggled against the impulse to burglarize and later on to kill. His attempts to fight the impulse produced anxiety, sweating and headaches. With the lipstick of one of the victims he wrote on the mirror, "Catch me before I kill again. I can't help myself." Eugene, a case described by Guttmacher[10], killed with a knife two 11-year-old girls while on parole, serving a sentence for attacking several women with a penknife. The sexual nature of his attacks apparently had not been recognized by the court and he was treated like a common criminal just serving a sentence for assault.

One of the New Jersey cases was examined at the state Diagnostic Center by Doctor Ralph Brancale five years prior to the murder of the victim. He was known then to have perpetrated the following acts: he set fires, he cut his mother's underclothes, he broke into a neighbor's house and wrecked several rooms. A year after this examination, he molested two little girls and stuffed cleansing tissue in their mouths. While the sex murders in Group 1 are of compulsive nature, and very likely more murders or assaults will be perpetrated if the murderer is not apprehended, the murders in Group 2 are basically accidental and usually committed in a state of frustration, fear and anger connected with the offender's inability to perform the sexual act or with his feelings or impotence and inadequacy. The following case examined by the author in one of the New Jersey prisons will illustrate this mechanism:

Case 1

A 40-year-old, unmarried, weak, inadequate chronic alcoholic with a deep feeling of inferiority and with potency disturbances, was drinking with his friend in a tavern. There they met a woman who agreed to follow both men into their car. She refused to have sex relations. He hit her head and body with his fist. When she lost consciousness, both men took her to a motel and put her to bed. The offender climbed on top of her and attempted intercourse but was unable to obtain an erection. He fell asleep. He found her dead the next morning, and turned himself in to the authorities.

Another case examined by the author at the Diagnostic Center illustrates the influence of fear in sex murders belonging to Group 2:

Case 2

A 14-year-old boy attempted intercourse with a six-year-old girl. Since he could not effect penetration, he forcibly proceeded to have anal intercourse. The girl fainted. He became frightened and hid her in a pile of automobile tires where she died from asphyxiation.

Group 3 can be best illustrated by the following case:

Case 3

A 40-year-old single male, an inmate of one of the New Jersey prisons, was serving a sentence for assault and battery at the time of the examination. He had clubbed a young woman on the street. He pulled her into his car. Her screams brought rescue so that he was forced to run away. Upon arrest the police found in his room and in his car blackjacks, a knife, a rifle, a noose, pornographic pictures, and a volume of *Psychopathis Sexualis* by Krafft-Ebing. He had a good army and work record, and was never arrested prior to the offense. He did not drink and, in general, enjoyed a good reputation. He said that the girl had been clubbed in an attempt at robbery. Under sodium amobarbital injected intravenously he revealed the following:

At the age of nine years he tied a little girl's legs. When she screamed and kicked he experienced a "peculiar thrill." Since then, he has always been thrilled by pictures or motion pictures in which women were tied by savages in the jungle. He frequently fantasized about tying women's legs. He satisfied his urge just by looking at porno-graphic pictures. While in service, he corresponded with a girl whom he intended to marry. After discharge, he disrupted the relationship, rationalizing his celibacy by the duty to support his aged mother. Although he associated with others, he basically was withdrawn and had a feeling of loneliness and isolation. Under sodium amobarbital he said the following: "I tied her legs because I wanted to feel that she was my own, that she was close to me. I don't want to hurt people (cries bitterly). During the robbery, I wanted to hit a girl's head, and at the same time I wanted to soften the hitting, since I didn't want to hurt her (cries). I was scared, I was afraid that I'd hurt her."

There is evidence in the literature that simple assaults on women may presage sexual killing. To illustrate this view, I will cite shortly several cases. (1) Eugene . . . described by Guttmacher[10] assaulted women with a knife prior to stabbing to death two little girls. (2) Roche, arrested in New York City for inflicting stab wounds on a 14-year old girl, had at the time a record for five murders. According to the newspaper reports he said "sex entered his life when he was sixteen and that he forced himself on girls with a knife." (3) Bruno . . . described by Magnus Hirschfield[11] impulsively choked a prostitute to death. While she was lying inert, he attempted intercourse with the corpse, but could not obtain an erection. He then stabbed the body and later proceeded to choke the victim's mother. Prior to this crime, he grabbed another woman by the throat, but when she fell to the ground he became terrified and asked her forgiveness. One of the sex murders committed recently in New Jersey by an 18-year old boy was preceded by assaulting two little girls, stuffing their mouths with tissue paper as well as destruction of female clothing. In the other sex murder case, committed by a 23-year-old male, his history shows that at the age of 14 years he threw a nine-year old girl to the ground, exposed himself and attempted sodomy. Case 3 reported above, tied little girls' legs at the age of nine years and has frequently phantasied about it since then. The list of such incidents preceding murder is impressive. This, however, poses a very serious prognostic problem since incidents of sudden unprovoked assault on women, or sadistic phantasies, are fortunately more frequent that the ultimate murder. The following case will illustrate the responsibility of a psychiatrist when he is called to examine this type of behavior.

Case 4

A thirty-five-year-old male was serving a short prison term for larceny. Consultation was requested since the custodial officers found, in his cell, drawings of torture and murder of women in medieval dungeons, as well as hundreds of scribbled pages of horror stories, all products of his own genius. A sample of his writings will illustrate the extent of his sadistic phantasies: "A naked man hung swinging and writhing his genitals. Next to him hung a plump woman who had cords threaded through her breasts and she was hanging by them. The weight of her body pulled them up by her face. It was a pitiful sight as she writhed and squirmed. The mob was jabbing sticks at her buttocks and vagina while she hung there writhing."

The prison authorities wanted a prognosis of this man's behavior.

He obviously has sadistic phantasies, his personality was somewhat disorganized and characterized by schizoid traits. Yet, there was no history of violence of any kind. In another case, a 16-year-old boy surrendered to the police saying he was afraid he would choke his girlfriend. It appeared during a sodium amobarbital interview that he made several such attempts and that he frequently phantasied of seeing his mother dead in a coffin. He was failing in school, and felt lonely, isolated, and rejected.

Another 17-year-old boy fell asleep riding the bus, and when he woke up he found himself at the end of the line. A young woman descended with him and, when both crossed the street, he suddenly struck her and threw her down without provocation.

Shall we commit all these cases as potential sex murderers? Have we enough data to predict sexual murders? The answer is no. The best we can do is to be suspicious of such a possibility. Much more coordinated clinical research in the field is necessary. Unfortunately, most of the cases, although reported in the press, are not thoroughly examined and reported in the professional literature.

Prognosis should be based on a combination of (1) history of assaults on women or girls, (2) dislike and resentment of the opposite sex, (3) sadistic phantasies, (4) sexual preoccupations, particularly fetishism of female underclothing, and (5) schizoid traits or a well-defined schizophrenic process. Undoubtedly, many of the sex murderers reported in the press and in the literature are well-integrated paranoid schizophrenics who do not impress many examiners as being psychotic. As far as the psychodynamic factors leading to sexual violence are concerned, it is my opinion that in cases belonging to Groups 1, 3, and 4, there is a resentment of the maternal figure transferred to womanhood in general. The following case illustrates this point.

Case 5

A 26-year-old male picked up a 45-year-old woman in a tavern, took her in his car and drove to an isolated place. Both undressed and, after completing intercourse, she told him she was supposed to go to the hospital for a checkup. It flashed through his mind that his mother had just come home from the hospital. He then suddenly put his hands on her neck and with the words, "Go and die there, bitch," he strangled her. On projective tests, he referred to women as "whores." He also revealed repetitive dreams of chasing naked women up a tree and of being the master of a "whorehouse." A great deal of hostility to his mother was also expressed. This man was a panty fetishist. He bragged of having collected 185 pairs.

Davidson[7] says that there is some evidence that public clamor, gruesome and sadistic pictures, as well as newspaper reports, may stimulate sadistic acts. Gilles de Ray of France, executed in 1440 for murder and mutilation of 800 children, said that he was stimulated by the accounts of orgies of the Roman emperors[8]. In my own experience at least two individuals reported here asserted that they were stimulated by pictures and horror stories.

SUMMARY AND CONCLUSIONS

Extreme manifestations of sexual violence are relatively rare. The majority of sex offenders commit minor crimes of a nonaggressive nature. There are four types of sexual violence:

1. Murder is a prerequisite of sexual satisfaction.
2. Murder is committed in a state of fear or anger connected with frustration.
3. Sexual satisfaction is connected with aggressive acts against women such as stabbing, clubbing or choking.
4. Sadistic needs are expressed in phantasy only. There is evidence that many instances of compulsive sexual murders were preceded by manifestations belonging to Type 3.

Prognosis is difficult, and not enough detailed studies are available. A combination of aggressive acts against women, hatred of the opposite sex, hostility for maternal figures, sexual preoccupations, and schizoid traits should alert the examining physician to the possibility of sexual murder in the future. These traits or acts should not be dismissed lightly even when performed by children.

When one encounters an adolescent with all these factors, unless he is manifestly psychotic, there will be reluctance to deprive him indefinitely of liberty, since no one can be certain that such an act will be committed. If no crime is committed, they will not be accepted by penal institutions. If they are not notoriously psychotic, they will not be kept in mental hospitals. Institutional treatment of suspects is not available and the value and limitations of psychotherapy has not been evaluated yet. Karpman[4] asserts that no sex murderer has even been analyzed. Besides, the family of the suspects may be unable to afford, or unwilling to accept, private or clinic treatment. The patient may live too far away from the nearest clinic or clinic facilities may be insufficient.

Public clamor to do something about this can be satisfied only in the following ways: (a) More clinical research, (b) more exchange of information through publication in scientific papers of cases that come under the attention of psychiatrists, (c) impressing upon courts the necessity to refer for psychiatric examination all the cases of compulsive assaults on women, and (d) the family physician's understanding that he should not dismiss violence of children against girls, particularly when it is connected with sexual preoccupations as childish pranks; instead he/she should request a psychiatric consultation.

REFERENCES

1. Brancale, R., Ellis, A. & Doorbar, R. (1952). Psychiatric and psychological investigating of convicted sex offenders. *American Journal of Psychiatry, 109*:17.
2. Ellis, A. & Brancale, R. (1956). *The psychology of sex offenders.* Springfield, IL: Charles C Thomas.
3. Brancale, Ralph (1956). Personal communication.
4. Karpman, B. (1954). *The sexual offender and his offenses,* New York: Julian Press.
5. Brancale, Ralph: Personal communication, 1956.
6. Rogers, E & Weiss, J. (1954). *California Sexual Deviation Research, State of California Department of Mental Hygiene.* Sacramento, CA.
7. Davidson, H. (1952). *Forensic psychiatry.* New York: Donald Press.
8. Krafft-Ebing, R. von: *Psychopathia sexualis.* Translated by Gar Nicht. Physicians and Surgeons Book Company, Brooklyn, New York, 1934 (originally published, 1886).
9. Freeman, L. (1956). *Before I kill again.* New York: Pocket Books, Inc.
10. Guttmacher, M. S. (1954). *Sex offenses: The problem, causes and prevention.* New York: Norton.
11. Hirschfield, M. (1940). *Sexual anomalies and perversions.* New York: Emerson Books.

Chapter 2

EXTREME MANIFESTATIONS OF SEXUAL AGGRESSION

The experience with more than 5,500 sex offenders examined at the New Jersey State Diagnostic Center under the purview of the New Jersey Sex Law confirmed the initial findings by Brancale et al.[1] These authors found the majority of the cases are "innocuous, inadequate, passive and minor sex offenders rather than sadistic fiends." Only 4.5 percent of the first 1,206 cases seen at the Diagnostic Center were sentences for rape.[2] The sexual nature of unprovoked assaults and the murder of females by males frequently is not recognized by the arresting or sentencing authorities because of the absence of manifest sexual motivation or activity. In fact, the offender may rationalize his offense by presenting it as a common crime such as robbery. A case previously reported[3] admitted to an attempted robbery in explaining his unprovoked blackjack attack on a young woman. Under the influence of intravenously injected sodium amytal, it became evident that he was motivated by abnormal sexual urges and by a compulsive need to tie female legs.

A recent newspaper account indicates, in the following words, how a repetitive, dangerous, sexually motivated pattern was treated in a similar way: "A 21-year-old ex-convict . . . who terrorized residents of . . . last December with a series of knife attacks on women was sent to . . . reformatory. He pleaded guilty to two robbery indictments but the judge ignored the plea and cited the previous record noting that he had been discharged from the Air Force for assaulting a woman." It is clear that the majority of those offenders do not qualify under sex law and

---

Source: Revitch, E. (1965). Extreme Manifestations of Sexual Aggression. *The Welfare Reporter, 16*:10-16.

therefore most of them are not referred to the Diagnostic Center for presentence evaluation. I was able to collect 43 cases of unprovoked assaults, nine of which resulted in murder. Most of these cases were examined at the New Jersey State Diagnostic Center and in the New Jersey prison system. Some came to my attention through private referrals and one case I examined in an Army General Hospital during World War II. He was then a 19-year-old private, who since the age of 12 years, had a compulsive need to break into a house and to hit a sleeping woman with a brick. Battery with a heavy object, choking the victim, or inflicting multiple knife stab wounds was the most common method of attack seen in our case material. Cannibalism, drinking or victim's blood, evisceration and extreme mutilation of the body reported by the classical authors[4,5] was not observed in our case material.

Genital manifestations such as erection and ejaculation may accompany the aggressive acts but are not necessarily present. In some cases, the assaults are of a compelling nature and are committed in a repetitive, ritualistic manner on females with specific attributes. The urge to attack may be so overpowering that the offender experiences severe anxiety unless he abstains. Thus, Krafft-Ebing[4] in reporting the case of a patient who stabbed a woman in the genitals wrote: "for a while he succeeded in mastering his morbid cravings, but this produced feelings of anxiety and a copious perspiration would break out from his entire body." In other cases, the assaults may be repetitive but without the ritualistic pattern of attack or choice of victim. In fact, cases of multiple attacks on men, women and children are known, the classical example being that of Peter Kurten.[6] At the age of nine years, Kurten pushed a boy off a raft; at 16 he attempted to choke a girl; at 17 he attempted to shoot another girl; at 18 he attacked women physically. Later in life, he committed numerous murders of men, women and children, badly mutilating the victims' bodies. On one occasion, unable to find a human victim, he killed a swan and drank the bird's blood.

In another variety of cases, the need to attack is not compelling but is stimulated by a frustrating event challenging the attacker's self-concept as a male. The best example is beating or murder of the victim during an unsuccessful attempt to have intercourse, or to rape, because of potency failure. Sometimes the attack represents a release of accumulated tensions described by Wertham under the name catathymic crisis.[7] The victim is usually known to the offender. Her very presence, and what the attacker interprets as seductiveness causes tension, anxiety, brooding and finally a need to destroy the source of the turmoil. This need may, at first, be perceived as a vague fantasy but then, little by little, it takes hold of the potential attacker, and finally in spite of an inner struggle and seeking help, the act is performed and relief from turmoil obtained. A case illustrating this mechanism is that of a 22-year-old man who killed his girlfriend with numerous stab wounds during a car ride. For several months prior to the event, he had vague thoughts of killing her and he sought help against the impulse in contacting a friend and his minister. As it is usual in these cases, his thoughts were vague and seemed unrealistic and fantastic, not only to others but also to himself. After the murder, he surrendered to the State Police. In the interview he was less concerned with murder than with the "sin" of sexual relations with his girlfriend. He quoted the scriptures and compared his act with that of Abraham's sacrifice of Isaac. He was angered by the prosecutors' theory of premeditation and planning. "They all just think that I planned it, it was just in my mind. I never thought it would happen. I never really meant it."

The pretrial psychiatric examination of these offenders usually degenerates into the sane-insane issue. A review of the various newspaper accounts and of cases reported in literature shows the predominance of a schizoid pattern and of overt clinical schizophrenic psychosis, even in cases determined by the jury to be sane. In our material, only ten cases could be qualified under the category of a personality pattern disturbance, while the rest were either overtly schizophrenic or schizoid. Guttmacher[8] deplores the failure to recognize the aggressive sexual motivation, and possibly the repetitive pattern in this type of offense and he recommends the adoption of Article 3, paragraph 5, of the Model Sentencing Act which takes into consideration the dangerousness of the offender.

A great deal of experience in criminological aspects of psychiatry is necessary in order to give a nearly reliable dynamic and prognostic evaluation of the offender. Therefore, should the Model Sentencing Act be adopted in our state, it would seem unfair to qualify an offender as dangerous without a challenge or confirmation by another expert or by a board of experts. With these considerations in view, I made an attempt to elicit clinical manifestations and dynamic factors which could be useful as prognostic signs in cases under study.[9] Hatred of women and preoccupation with sexual mortality are most commonly found either in direct interviews or under the influence of intravenously injected sodium amytal and in responses to the TAT. In the younger preadolescent and adolescent group, preoccupation with sexual mortality and particularly with fancied, implied, or overt sexual misconduct and seductiveness of mother, or mother surrogate, seems to be the dominant factor. In the older group, hatred for women seems to be stressed to a greater extent. A newspaper account of a thirty-six-year-old trucker's helper who had strangled four women illustrates this phenomenon, "he nursed a grudge against all women for the past 21 years."

Maternal overprotection and seductiveness, ambivalent feelings toward the son, and his outright infantilization and effeminization by the mother are frequently uncovered in just a few interviews. The extrapolation from these findings leads us to believe that the generally accepted theory of incestuous conflicts is the best explanation of the offender's behavior. The female victim is then a maternal symbol, a scapegoat for the offender's mother. In fact, some of our cases attacked females shortly after an argument with mother or sister. In one case an adolescent boy strangled two women shortly after such an argument.

Minor sexual offenses which are usually referred under the provisions of Sex Act to the New Jersey State Diagnostic Center are rare in the history of attackers. This finding was confirmed by Guttmacher.[8] Burglaries committed solo and under bizarre circumstances, fetishism of female undergarments, repetitive or isolated assaults on females, and aggressive, sadistic fantasies revealed either through responses to the TAT or through more direct interview techniques seem to be of important prognostic significance. Even greater prognostic significance is noted if these signs are connected with hostility to women, and various preoccupations involving mother's sexuality, along with the presence of schizoid features or clinical schizophrenia.

Case 1

This case is presented to illustrate the early onset of sexually aggressive acts, the dynamic factors underlying it, and our failure to deal effectively with such conditions even when discovered in early childhood. The patient, then an 11-year-old boy, was admitted to the New Jersey State Diagnostic Center for in-patient evaluation of several attempts to choke little girls. The boy's father deserted the family and his whereabouts were unknown. His mother was sentenced to the reformatory for women for neglect of her children, and she was known to be sexually promiscuous. The boy was only in second grade at the time of the examination. His IQ on the Wechsler Bellevue Intelligence Test was 72. A report from a mental hygiene clinic indicated that the boy's mother had little concern for him. The psychiatric interviews under intravenously injected sodium amytal revealed excessive masturbation with fantasies of incestuous relations with his mother. There were memories of witnessing the mother's promiscuous behavior with various men. He saw his mother as rejecting and "bad," and he repeatedly expressed a desire to read the Bible since the Bible was "good." As far as the victims of his offenses were concerned, at first he expressed a feeling of being slighted by them, but in the deeper stages of narcosis he mumbled the choking of the girls made him feel "glad." In the initial stages of the interview, he sang songs with a pornographic content involving his parents. While at the Diagnostic Center, a great deal of sexual preoccupation and homosexual attempts were reported by the ward personnel.

COMMENT. These children present a serious disposition problem since they are in dire need of institutional placement with special treatment facilities. As an expedience, they are transferred to the State Home for Boys since other facilities are usually unavailable and since they are too disturbed to be placed in foster homes.

Case 2

A 14-year-old boy was referred by the juvenile court to the New Jersey State Diagnostic Center for choking, beating and stabbing a 10-year-old girl who came to his house to visit the boy's sister. The psychometric tests revealed normal intelligence. He was a sickly child, disinterested in sports and somewhat withdrawn. His hobby was nature studies. He recollected the incident in the following words: "When I heard her knocking at the door, my stomach was all upset, my mouth was dry and my head was spinning all around. Then I remembered calling her in. Then I took the knife and I attacked her, choked her and cut her neck. Then I awoke like from a dream and let her go. Then I went to my room and I prayed." He expressed a dislike for all girls and he complained that some girls in school made fun of him. He knew practically nothing about sex and he never danced or kissed a girl. The victim of the offence was a frequent visitor to the house and, according to the boy's sister, she liked him. A few hours prior to the incident he had an argument with his mother since she inadvertently had broken one of his specimens. In another interview under hypnosis, he revealed preoccupations with his body shape and his sensitivity over being poor in shows of masculinity such as in ball games. He recollected the various incidents of avoiding girls' presence, and he revealed fantasies of maternal purity and absence of sexual relations between parents since "it is forbidden." He also claimed he would avoid a girl with indecent behavior.

COMMENT. In this case, schizoid characteristics are combined with hostility to females, with preoccupations with sexual morality, and with his own defective male image. An argument with the mother precipitated the attack. The question of prognosis is of great importance. A review of similar cases shows the possibility of a repetitive pattern. The question of whether a boy like this should be institutionalized, or whether he can be treated outside on an out-patient basis, is of great significance and cannot be decided in a rule of thumb manner.

Case 3

This patient was first examined by the author at the age of fourteen years for an unprovoked attack and choking of a six-year-old girl. The attack took place after an argument with his sister. Already at that time, he was known to be a female undergarment fetishist and he was known to the police to steal female bathing suits and girdles from the clotheslines. On psychometric tests, he demonstrated a normal intelligence while the projective tests revealed confusion in sexual role identification and a conflictual relationship with his mother. I then considered him to harbor a dangerous potential, and I recommended reevaluation on an in-patient basis. The parents objected considering his behavior just a juvenile prank. The boy returned to the Diagnostic Center six years later under the provisions of the New Jersey Sex Law for evaluation of the offense of carnal abuse, and indecent assault which consisted in sexual play with a nine-year-old girl. Between the two appearances he had two short jail sentences for larceny.

He revealed family tensions not disclosed by the parents six years previously. He also admitted to the loss of his driver's license in several states because of 17 accidents. Due to the special interest in this case, I requested reexamination under the influence of intravenously injected sodium amytal. This was done three weeks later. Hostility toward women was revealed in the following statements: "Women are no damn good," or "I am a friend to everybody . . . but women think they are the bosses. They are no good." He also revealed fantasies of himself becoming a girl in order to wear female clothing. He revealed a strange fantasy of police officers being castrated so they could not have sex relations with females they may arrest. In his masturbatory fantasies he visualized sexual relations with his sister and his mother, and at the same time, he revealed fear of intercourse. In deeper stages of narcosis, he spoke about "hitting women . . . I could smash a lot of them. . . . Many times I felt like slapping my girlfriend. I told Pat to take off her bathing suit or I'd kill her. She took the bathing suit off, but I did nothing." At times with Pat in his car, he drove ninety miles an hour in order to kill Pat since, "if I kill her she becomes mine, then no one else could have her." He also spoke about having a knife in his car in order to kill Pat, and that sex and killing seemed identical to him.

COMMENT. Whereas I was unable to recommend anything of value when I saw the patient in his adolescence, I was now able to recommend placement under the purview of the Sex Act and have him thus committed to a State Hospital. Had he committed another crime of a nonsexual nature or more correctly not considered sexual such as attack with a knife or attempt to choke, he would just serve a short prison sentence and then continue with more dangerous assaults after release.

DISCUSSION

The problem of prognosis and disposition constantly confronts us at the Diagnostic Center. Since most of the cases referred for evaluation do not belong to the well-defined area described in the classical text books in psychiatry, we are thus threading in a virgin and unchartered territory. The prognostic evaluations and recommendations will be more subjective than in cases belonging to better known and defined diagnostic categories. Ewalt[10] stated in his presidential address at the 1964 annual meeting of the American Psychiatric Association that in such cases, the psychiatrist "is on shaky ground when he attempts to predict future behavior under unspecified circumstances, [but] as psychiatrists, we are prepared by training and experience in interpreting, predicting, and modifying human behavior, and it is our responsibility to help as much as we can while we are aware of our limitations."

The increasing population and the rapidly changing conditions of life defy simple solutions. Newer and newer problems are brought into focus for which old solutions are inapplicable, and problems still requiring the older solutions are so great in number the facilities available are insufficient to cope with them. I believe that this is what Commissioner Lloyd McCorkle meant in his paper presented to the 1964 annual meeting of the New Jersey Medical Society.[11] The dangerous sexual aggressions and the potential sex murderers should be viewed as an isolated and not too common case in the array of behavioral problems.

In essence, the problem is that of the recognition and disposition of dangerous offenders. Too often, transfer to the State Home for Boys is resorted to as an expedient for lack of other facilities. It is obvious that such a commitment in Case 1 will not safeguard the potential victim at some future date. In another case of a youthful sex murder of a little girl, it was necessary to commit him to the State Home for Boys since in spite of his low IQ of 72, he was not considered eligible for an institution for mentally defectives. The youth came from a disorganized background with an inadequate, alcoholic father and with a mother who deserted the family. After release from the State Home, he will return to a broken family, living in a congested, delinquent area.

In case of murder by an adult, the problem of prevention is solved through legal means. However, in case of minor attacks by a potential murderer or recidivist, the law has no way to deal with the offender other than to give an appropriate prison sentence, which sooner or later ends in release without an attempt to treat or modify the behavior. In one of our cases, more dangerous and overtly homicidal activities took place after termination of the sentence. Many of these offenders have enough pathology to have them committed to the Vroom Building as criminally insane. Unfortunately, the public still believes that more protection will be afforded by imprisonment rather than by indefinite hospital commitment. In cases of potentially dangerous aggressions by children or adolescents, the warning is not taken into consideration by parents and at times by the court. Thus, nothing was done for Case 3 after his evaluation during adolescence. A case of an offender, at the age of thirteen years, was also left alone until, at the age of 19, he attacked and strangled a female schoolmate. Yet, sufficient warning was given to the parents.

Wertham[7] requested the commutation of the death sentence of the well-known case of Albert Fish, and urged the Governor "to make this case an example and starting point for real scrutiny of the whole haphazard and bureaucratic chaos of the psychiatric prevention of violent crimes." It would be naïve to expect easy answers and easy solutions to complex problems. It should be the purpose of the Diagnostic Center, and of similar institutions, to accumulate experience and to give recommendations on the basis of these studies. It is up to the judiciary to review the findings and recommendations and, together with the psychiatrists involved in this work, to search for new ways of prevention and safeguards. I suspect that no final solution will ever be found, at least in the foreseeable future. Yet, without attempts to do so, the present day dispositions will become more and more anachronistic as time marches on.

REFERENCES

1. Brancale, R., Ellis, A., Doorbar, R. (1952). Psychiatric and psychological investigations of convicted sex offenders. *American Journal of Psychiatry, 109*:17.
2. Brancale, R., Vuocolo, A., MacNeil, D. (1969). *Diagnostic Center Report.* Unpublished Study.
3. Revitch, E. (1957). Sex Murder and Sex Aggression. *Journal of the Medical Society of New Jersey, 54*:519.
4. Krafft-Ebing. 1934, (originally published, 1886). *Psychopathia Sexualis,* Translated by F. J. Rebman. New York: Physicians and Surgeons Book Company.
5. Hirshfield, M. (1944). *Sexual anomalies and perversions.* London: Francis Aldor.
6. Wilson, C., Pitman, P. (1962). *Encyclopedia of murder.* New York: G. P. Putnam and Sons.
7. Wertham, F. (1949). *The show of violence.* New York: Eton Books, Inc.
8. Guttmacher, M. S. (1963). Dangerous offenders. *Crime and Delinquency, 9*:38.
9. Revitch, E. (May 20, 1964). Sex Murder and the Potential Sex Murderer in press) Read at 198th Annual Meeting of the New Jersey Medical Society, Atlantic City.
10. Ewalt, J. R. (May 4, 1964). Presidential Address: 120th Annual Meeting of the American Psychiatric Association, Los Angeles.
11. McCorkle, L. (May 20, 1964). Acknowledged but Unmet Needs. Read at the 198th Annual Meeting of the New Jersey Medical Society, Atlantic City.

Chapter 3

SEX MURDER AND THE POTENTIAL SEX MURDERER

It is intended in this paper to determine the dynamic factors involved in the crime of murder and unprovoked attacks on women by males, and find the possible clues for prediction of such an eventuality. A review of the literature[1-6] and newspaper accounts of 9 murders and 34 assaults, most of which were examined through association with the New Jersey Diagnostic Center, point to the following patterns. These attacks, with or without resulting deaths, are usually committed through pushing, choking, inflicting multiple knife wounds or battering the victim with a heavy object. A case of compulsive shooting of a female, and compulsive throwing of a female child off a roof, were found in the newspaper accounts. Evisceration, extreme mutilation of the body, cannibalism and drinking victim's blood reported in the literature were summarized in a previous paper.[7] Erection and ejaculation may or may not accompany the aggressive acts, while rape and attempted rape are infrequent, contrary to popular conception. The columnist Max Lerner[8] made these remarks: "In many cases of sexual brutality and murder, the act is never committed. Violence serves as a substitute for it."

Attacks and murders may be described by the police and the courts as attempts at robbery and theft or as assault and battery. The underlying sexual dynamics may be completely disregarded. In a case previously reported,8 a man arrested for assault with intent to rob had attacked a woman with a blackjack. He rationalized that he needed money and that a woman was the easier victim. Under intravenous

---

Source: Revitch, E. (1965). Sex murder and the potential sex murderer. *Diseases of the Nervous System, 26*:640-648.

sodium amytal he revealed long-standing fantasies of tying female legs and said that this was the purpose of his attack. A noose, a rifle, and the book *Psychopathia Sexualis* found in his car were not considered clues. Only in isolated instances were these cases examined as sex offenders.

In more than 5,000 cases referred to the Diagnostic Center, the findings of Brancale et al.[9] indicate that the majority of sex offenders are "innocuous, inadequate, passive and minor offenders rather than violent sadistic sex fiends." Only 4.5 percent of the first 1,206 cases[10] were charged with rape. The majority of the offenses consisted of indecent exposure, homosexual relations, obscene phone calls, dissemination of obscene literature, and sexual relations with the consent of juvenile partners below the age of 16 years. Of the offenses committed, 67 to 69 percent were against children, but these offenses were mostly of a noncoital and nonaggressive nature.[11] Aggressive acts causing bodily injury or death are very rare in comparison with the nonaggressive offenses.

CASE MATERIAL

Tables 3.1 through 3.5 summarize the characteristics of the 43 cases investigated in the present study.

Table 3.1
TYPE OF ATTACKS IN 43 CASES UNDER STUDY

Pushing The Victim	6
Battery	8
Choking	11
Knife Attacks	11
Unspecified	5
Threats, Battery, Abduction	2
Total (Including 9 Murders)	43

Table 3.2
CASES INVOLVING MURDER

Choking*	3
Suffocation of little girl during attempted rape.	2
Knife attacks.	3
Battery with a heavy object.	1

*One perpetrator choked two victims on the same day

Table 3.3
AGE DISTRIBUTION OF AGGRESSIVE OFFENDERS

AGE (YRS.)	NO.
11	1
12	3
14	8
15	5
16	2
17	6
18	2
19	4
20-25	5
26-30	2
30-35	2
35-40	3
Total	43

Table 3.4
AGE DISTRIBUTION OF 9 MURDER CASES

AGE (YRS.)	NO.
14	2
15	2
19	3
23	1
26	1

The large number of adolescents is due to the type of referrals. The court is more inclined to send an aggressive adolescent for an in-patient study than to refer an adult whose pathological motivation may be concealed.

Table 3.5
FULL SCALE WECHSLER-BELLEVUE IQ SCORES

IQ	NO.
43-72	5
80-90	3
90-110	14
110-120	3
Above 120	2
Total	27

IQ not available in 16 cases; eight patients had a physical deformity or were physically inadequate.

CLASSIFICATION AND NATURAL HISTORY

The following classification (which is a modification of that employed in an earlier paper[7]) is used in this study:

1. *Impulsive Murder and Assault.* Murder or assault are not in themselves required for satisfaction but are a consequence of fear, anger, or frustration over impotence or resistance of the victim during rape, attempted rape, or intercourse with the consent of the victim.
2. *Compulsive Murder and Assault.* Either murder or assault on a female is an expression of a compulsive need and provides satisfaction, with or without accompanying sexual manifestations such as erection and ejaculation. The assaults are usually repetitive and are frequently committed in a similar ritualistic manner.
3. *Catathymic Crisis.* Under the name of Catathymic Crisis, Wertham[12] described the release of accumulated tension: "a catathymic reaction is the transformation of the stream of thought, as the result of certain complexes of ideas, that are charged with a strong affect, usually a wish, a fear of an ambivalent striving." The accumulation of tension released through the attack may be of long duration, or it may be a displacement of suddenly induced hostile emotions from mother, or mother surrogate, to the victim.

Either a specific female known to the assailant, or one having specific attributes, will become a victim, or the victim may be chosen impersonally because of availability. In our material, 18 cases knew their victims while 25 did not. In categories 2 and 3, the offender may attempt to master his impulse and go through a period of doubt and brooding. Guttmacher[1] quotes Heirens as saying: "on one occasion I took off my clothes and thought if I did that I would not be able to get out. I got ready for bed. I resisted for about 2 hours. I tore sheets out of place and went into a sweat." Krafft-Ebing[3] in reporting the case of a 20-year-old male who stabbed girls in the genitals stated: "For awhile he succeeded in mastering his morbid cravings, but this produced feelings of anxiety, and perspiration would break out on his entire body." Minor attacks on women such as choking as if in jest, hitting, pinching, superficial cutting, etc., were reported in the literature, and seen in our series of cases, as ending either in serious assaults or in murder. The following cases from the literature may be used for illustration.

Bruno G.[2] attempted to choke a date, but after the attempt he apologized. Eventually, he choked a prostitute and her mother to death, and then attempted unsuccessfully to have sexual relations with the body of the younger victim. DeRivers' case[4] was known to have written threatening letters to a girl and to have slapped another girl prior to smashing his girlfriend's head with a hammer. The multiple sadistic murderer Peter Kurten[6] was known to have pushed a boy off a raft at the age of nine years, attempted to strangle a girl during intercourse at the age of 16 years, attempted to shoot a girl at the age of 17 years, and physically attacked women at the age of 18 years. After his arrest, many young women reported their experience of having been choked or mistreated by him during courtship and love-making. John F. Roche, who was accused of having committed five sadistic murders within a period of 19 months, "at age 16 forced himself upon girls with a knife" according to the newspaper accounts. Eugene,[1] after release from prison where he served a sentence for knife attacks on women, stabbed two young girls, one of whom died as a result of the wounds. Heath[13] mistreated and beat prostitutes in Cairo brothels prior to sadistic murders in England which finally led to his execution.

Thirty out of our 43 cases committed previous offenses. Only three of these prior offenses consisted of overt sexual offenses, while 12 consisted of breaking and entering. Guttmacher[14] brought up a similar experience of infrequent sexual offenses and of the importance of breaking and entering in the previous record of violent sex offenders. Four out of 12 cases combined breaking and entering with assault or threats to a female occupant. Fetishism of female underwear or lingerie was elicited in nine cases. The literature and newspaper accounts suggest the possibility of an intimate connection between fetishism of female underwear, breaking and entering, and assaults on women. A newspaper account of an 18-year-old student is illustrative. This young man slipped into an apartment at night, strangled an 18-year-old girl with a cord, and then he cut up her remains. He was known to prowl at night in search of women's underthings hanging on clotheslines. In a California strangulation murder of a mother and daughter, the newspaper reported, "The house had been burglarized last year of nightgowns, dresses, a woman's wristwatch and woman's underwear." Although the mystery of the crime has not been solved at this time, the relationship of the two events is at least suggestive.

William Heirens[6,15,16] was a panty fetishist who, at an early age, started burglarizing homes to obtain female underwear. At the age of 17, he murdered two women and a six-year-old girl. The act of breaking and entering was accompanied by overt sexual excitement, and thus its sexual nature was no longer in the realm of unconsciousness. A case of Brancale's[17] combined breaking and entering with female glove fetishism. This individual murdered one female after breaking into her house and was suspected of having committed other murders of females in the area. In 21 out of 43 of our cases, there was evidence of sadistic fantasies prior to the arrest or psychiatric examination. In some cases, the fantasies were elicited only under the influence of intravenous sodium amytal or during the administration of the Thematic Apperception Test.

Peter Kurten[6] was constantly obsessed with sadistic fantasies and these were necessary as a stimulus for successful intercourse with his wife. Case W. in De River's[4] material fantasied for years about killing and raping little girls until he sadistically murdered three female children. Even in cases of impulsive murder belonging to group one, a history of sadistic fantasies or acts may be elicited at times. Thus, Roland J.,[16] a mentally defective boy of 17 who strangled his seven-year-old sister during an attempt at intercourse, had been observed (5 years previously) pulling feathers out of live pigeons. One knife murder and one assault ended in setting fire to the victims in our case material. Only one case of attempted burning of the victim was found in the literature.6 A newspaper account describing a New Jersey strangulation murder of a 61-year-old woman in her bedroom, with subsequent fire-setting, is suggestive of a similar mechanism.

Dynamic Factors

The following factors seem to be interwoven in the dynamic fabric of the assaults: hostility to women, preoccupation with maternal sexual conduct, overt or covert incestuous preoccupation, guilt over and rejection of sex as impure, sexual inferiority, and occasionally a need to completely possess the victim or whatever she may represent. On superficial levels of investigation, hostility to women was the most outstanding factor found to dominate in 27 of the 43 cases. In dividing the offenders into preadolescent-adolescent group, and an adult group starting with the age of 18 years, it was found that the hostility factor was more prominent in the adult group, while the sexual preoccupation factor, particularly preoccupation with sexual behavior, was more prominent in the younger group.

A newspaper account illustrates the hostility to females factor: "A 36-year-old trucker's helper, who said he nursed a grudge against all women for the past 21 years, told police yesterday that he had strangled three women and a 15-year-old girl in the past two weeks." The case of Eugene, reported by Guttmacher,[1] expressed in various ways his dislike for women. He composed a song with a refrain, "The women do you wrong."

The transfer of affect from mother to females in general, or to a particular female, could be elicited in all the cases. Wertham[19] described a 17-year-old boy who stabbed his mother 31 times while she was asleep. The boy was chaste, he disliked all women, and he was preoccupied with his mother's sexual indiscretions. Wertham compared the boy's preoccupations with those of Hamlet and Orestes. Both Hamlet and Orestes were obsessed with their mother's infidelity, and both women finally died through the action of their sons. It has been my observation in work with adolescents, that boys seem to be more traumatized and affected by mother's sexual misconduct than girls are by their father's indiscretions. Maternal overprotection, overt or covert seduction, infantilization, or outright feminization of the boy fosters ambivalent feelings and hostility to mother, which is transferred to women in general. A common denominator behind all the enumerated factors leading to the transfer of hostility from mother, to womanhood in general, is believed to be the struggle with an attempt at rejection of repressed incestuous wishes. These wishes are stimulated by maternal overprotection, seductiveness, and sexual promiscuity. This may be coupled with either their father's brutality, weakness, or unavailability. Outright maternal rejection may create a need to possess her.

A few patients revealed, under sodium amytal, fantasies of killing in order to completely possess the body, since a lifeless or dead body is not threatening and can be possessed entirely. This factor is expressed in Oscar Wilde's *Ballad of Reading Gaol*, "for each man kills the thing he loves," and in Dostoyevsky's novel *Idiot*. One of the characters in Dostoyevsky's novel, Rogojine, stabs to death the woman he loves and then shares the wake with the competitor for her attentions. Projective tests frequently reveal sexual preoccupations and the conception of the mother figure and females as overpowering, dangerous and threatening. A story of violence by a male against a female on TAT card 13 MF is a common finding. Fire-setting to the victim, after the assault in one case, was interpreted as a purification ritual. The fire-setting to the body after murder in another case could not be clarified, but similar unconscious motivation was suspected. In most of the cases, the victims represented a dangerous stimulus that had to be destroyed or overpowered. At times, feelings of triumph and revenge followed the assault. Intense anger was the overpowering emotion leading to the attack on females immediately following some intense frustration by the mother, wife or sister. Under the surface of anger and hostility to females, the various combinations of other factors could be usually elicited. Hatred and mutilation of cats was also reported by some.

A history of isolated and unexplainable attacks on women was discovered in routine psychiatric evaluations. These cases were not included in the present study. One of these perpetrators was serving a prison sentence for repeated burglaries and robberies at the time of the examination. He reported an incident of suddenly attacking a woman with a stick, and the experience of a feeling of triumph when, in younger years, he killed and burned cats. Hatred for cats is not uncommon in examination of delinquent adolescents and symbolic relationships between cats and females is suggestive in many instances. The relationship of criminal acts with states of depression was described by Woddis.[20] In my experience, such a relationship is common in states of depression, dejection, and frustration of a psychogenic origin. However, I have not seen such a relationship in typical involutional or manic-depressive states.

Easson and Steinhilber[21] found in a study of adolescent murderers and potential murderers, that parents have stimulated the acts through permissive attitudes toward aggressiveness. This view is supported by experimental studies of Berkowitz[22] which indicate a positive relationship between aggressive acts and expectations to aggress. A relationship with mother's permissiveness was clearly seen in one of our cases of a knife murder and fire-setting.

Diagnostic Considerations

In reviewing the literature, one gains an impression that the great majority of reported sadistic acts were perpetrated by either overt or latent psychotics, with poor control and explosive breaks with reality. Vacher the Ripper[3] was manifestly a case of paranoid schizophrenia, with a history of hospitalization in an insane asylum for "persecution mania." Yet, the experts of his time declared him "sane" and a "common criminal."

In the case of Verzeni, Krafft-Ebing[3] quoted the experts as saying: "There was nothing in the past that would indicate a mental disorder," but in describing his personality the experts added: "His character was peculiar, he was silent and inclined to be solitary." In the case of John F. Roche, the newspapers reported the following: "Three psychiatrists found the 27-year-old plumber's helper sane and capable of standing trial," and "psychiatrists found Roche free of mental disorder and declared that in him the more primitive sadistic forces of murder, rape, etc. were mobilized into a habit pattern." A week later one read:

> The sullen defendant told his lawyer he would not cooperate with them, and throughout the day Roche sat expressionless in his seat in front of two prison guards, while prospective jurors were questioned, and shook his head negatively each time one of his attorneys tried to consult with him. Time after time he snarled short answers to questions but most of the day he just stared grimly. "Roche is not interested in the trial at all," said Mr. Murray. "Talking to him is like sticking pins into an iceberg."

It is interesting that another expert diagnosed Roche as a case of schizophrenia which aroused the anger of the court.

Introversive tendencies, feelings of isolation, detachment, and blurring of reality boundaries were the most common findings in our cases. In our material, 19 cases were considered schizoid or dynamically schizophrenic, and nine cases clinically schizophrenic; five cases were diagnosed as mentally defective, and only 10 cases could be classified in the category of personality pattern or personality trait disturbance. The psychiatric diagnoses are not precise, frequently overlap, and should be viewed on a continuum rather than as tightly fixed categories.

Prognostic Considerations

In the evaluation of minor nonaggressive sex offenses referred by the court, the possibility of repetitiveness, and of violence in the future, is of prime importance. The bulk of the sex offenders commit no violence, and only three out of our 43 cases had a record of previous sex offenses. In Guttmacher's[14] series of sexually aggressive offenders, only one case had a previous conviction for exhibitionism. Of greater importance for prediction of potential violence, with sexual motivation, seems to be the following combination of factors: unprovoked assaults on women particularly choking or stabbing; offenses of breaking and entering committed solo in bizarre circumstances; fetishism of female underclothing; expressions of hatred, contempt or fear of women; violence against animals particularly violence against cats; violent and primitive fantasy life; confusion of sexual identity as elicited on projective tests; sexual inhibitions and moral preoccupations concerning sexual conduct; emotional shallowness and feelings of isolation and blurring of reality boundaries. In some of the cases, assaults were justified by the offenders on the basis of the victim's alleged immorality. In connection with this, it may be more than pure accident that prostitutes are not uncommonly the victims. Some of the prognostic factors reported here were also found by Satten et al.[23] in their cases of motiveless murder.

Disposition and Recommendations

According to Karpman,[5] no sex murderer has ever been psychoanalyzed. Psychotherapy of these offenders in a prison environment was attempted and described by Williams.[24] There are no effective short cut methods of treatment and a "methodical and patient working through of the transference is necessary."[24] It is not certain how many offenders were under treatment prior to or during the commitment of the offense. A case examined by Brancale[17] committed at least one murder while undergoing psychotherapy and close psychiatric supervision. The problem of therapy will not be discussed because of an absence of experience and documentation in the literature.

The main concern is the protection of the public. It is unfortunate that in most cases there is no social machinery for complete protection unless a crime is committed and the offender apprehended. In an assault without serious bodily injury, the offender is released at the end of his sentence, or he may be committed for a short time to a mental hospital and then released to continue the assaults and perhaps murder. Albert Fish[25] was briefly confined to a mental hospital and released without anyone being aware of his sadistic fantasies and exploits. Guttmacher[14] reported the case of a 40-year-old male released from prison after serving a sentence for murder and mutilation of a prostitute; 13 years later he served an 18-month sentence for threatening a prostitute with a knife; three years later he killed and beheaded another prostitute. In Guttmacher's words, "here was a murder that could be and should have been prevented by proper legal action."

In a local newspaper there was this item: "Ex-convict sentenced for knife attacks: A 21-year-old ex-convict from South Carolina who terrorized residents last December, with a series of knife attacks on women, was sent to the reformatory." The offender pleaded guilty to two robbery indictments, but "the judge ignored the plea and cited the offender's previous record, noting that he had been discharged from the Air Force for assaulting a woman." Not robbery, but compulsive pathological sexuality, was at the bottom of this person's attacks, and future assaults after release are at least possible.

Wertham,[25] in requesting commutation of the death sentence of Albert Fish, urged the governor "to make this case an example and starting point for real scrutiny of the whole haphazard and bureaucratic chaos of the psychiatric prevention of violent crimes." Article 3, paragraph 5, of the Model Sentencing Act considers the risk with the defendant, and recommends 30-year correctional treatment or custody if required for the protection of the public.

Unfortunately, psychiatrists without experience in this specific field are not acquainted with the natural history and prognostic factors of these dangerous offenders. Therefore, a sufficient contact with criminological aspects of psychiatry should be a must in residency training programs. Should the Model Sentencing Act or a modification be followed, the presentencing determination of the dangerousness of offenders will have to be evaluated in specialized institutions, by psychiatrists thoroughly experienced in this field. Perhaps a review by a board of psychiatrists, chosen by the defense, will minimize mistaken evaluations or personal factors. Complete and objective studies, and the results of projective tests with these cases, are seldom reported in the psychiatric literature, but sensational and emotionally laden descriptions of gruesome murders and assaults abound in public reporting. Unfortunately, many of these cases are only summarily examined in jail by the expert witnesses for defense and prosecution, and the result is no more than the legal verbiage about the "sane-insane" issue.

Further longitudinal clinical studies, exchange of information, special instruction in criminological psychiatry, specialized diagnostic centers, and adoption of the Model Sentencing Act, or its modification, are essential for public protection and eventually a possible cure of the offender.

SUMMARY

This paper deals with unprovoked violence and murder committed by males against females. The underlying sexual dynamics are frequently unrecognized. A review of the literature, newspaper accounts, and 34 assaults and nine murders examined by the author, indicate that choking, multiple knife stabs, and battery with a heavy object, are the most common methods of attack. Evisceration, severe mutilation, and cannibalism were reported in the literature. Fetishism of female underwear, previous offenses of breaking and entering committed solo and under bizarre circumstances, sadistic fantasies, minor assaults on females, and mutilation of animals are important prognostic signs. The more usual sexual offenses of a passive and nonaggressive nature are rare in the history of these offenders. Ambivalence to mother, preoccupation with sexual morality, and hatred of females, are the main dynamic factors. Maternal seductiveness and rejection, and father's unavailability, are the main etiological factors. Schizophrenia and schizoid personality are the most common diagnostic categories characterizing these cases. Adoption of the Model Sentencing Act concerning dangerous offenders and establishment of special diagnostic facilities, are recommended.

CASE HISTORIES

Case 1

This case is illustrative of the mechanisms involved in impulsive attacks. The patient was a 16-year-old referred for parole evaluation. At the age of 13, he had attempted sexual relations with a six-year-old girl by threats and coercion. This ended when he obtained an orgasm, but by that time the child was unconscious and seemed dead. He hid her under a pile of tires which caused the child's death by suffocation. The 16-year-old boy was from a broken family at a low socioeconomic level. In school he was withdrawn but worked to his capacity. He scored a Full Scale IQ of 70 on Wechsler–Bellevue Test. On projective tests, sexual preoccupation and sadistic, destructive fantasies were uncovered. On several Rorschach cards, he saw "some part of a woman," "inside of a woman," "intestines" and various parts of a female body. In a mild hypnotic trance, he revealed a memory of seeing his mother having sexual relations with a man, and he said he felt so unhappy that he wanted to knife the man. Under intravenous sodium amytal and methedrine, he spoke about homicidal anger and threats to kill his sister, fellow inmates, and the warden of the reformatory. He also recollected hitting his mother and slapping his sister.

DISCUSSION. On the surface, it would appear that the murder was due to fright or frustration. Yet, under amytal and methedrine medication, he revealed homicidal fantasies and anger; on the projective tests he saw female sex organs and dismembered female bodies. This case, as well as other similar cases, shows that even in incidental situational sex murders, underlying sadistic fantasies or needs may be elicited.

Case 2

This patient was examined at the Diagnostic Center as an in-patient at the age of 16 years, and again as an out-patient at 17, 21, and 24 years of age. The first episode which brought him to the attention of the authorities consisted of following a girl on the street and striking her on the head with a stick. In the psychiatric interview, he said, "I was mad at the whole female race. I was mad at all females and did not care which one I hit." This incident followed an argument with his sister. In the second episode, he followed a woman to her home, looked through the window and masturbated. He returned to the same place at night and threw a stone through the window. At the age of 21, he was re-examined because of indecent communications to females.

During the five-year interval between the two examinations, he spent 20 months in a juvenile institution, and then he served short jail sentences, and another reformatory sentence for touching sales girls in stores and for acts of voyeurism. Four months after release from the reformatory, he entered an apartment through a window and struck a young woman, sleeping in her bed, on the head with a pipe. Fortunately, the woman did not die.

In the psychiatric interviews, he seemed to be an unimpressive looking, weakly built, dilapidated young man with a stooped posture and flattened chest. He was emotionally flat but he spoke spontaneously without an attempt to minimize the offenses or to rationalize. Feelings of isolation, emptiness and dejection were elicited. In a superficial hypnotic trance, he revealed that other prisoners in jail called him "Oswald" and "Nazi." He liked to read stories about Nazi atrocities and regretted that he could not participate in concentration camp brutalities. In imagining himself as an S.S. officer, he said, "I would rape, I would beat both men and women if I didn't like them." He also spoke about burning people in ovens and seeing them "squirm." He imagined women as slaves and "if they don't do what I want them to, I would kill them." He also imagined himself a conqueror, killing female hostages from subdued countries if they disobeyed. He recollected that in childhood he was small, and "everyone made fun of me. I figured if I belonged to a country like Germany, I would be one of the big bosses and get even with all of them." He also had fantasies of being accepted and liked by women.

While peeping through the windows and masturbating, he fantasized that the female occupants will undress naked and invite him in. He attempted intercourse with prostitutes but he always had potency disturbances and the contacts ended with pushing the girls away in disgust. He was particularly angered with the necessity to pay a prostitute. "While breaking into a house, I would not have to pay and I would feel that the girl wanted me." Normally he felt shy with girls and even refused to share car rides with females to and from his place of employment. In the background, there is a history of parental discord, violence and rejection. He recollected that when his mother found out he had stolen some money from her, she put a sign on him, "I am a thief," and forced him to walk with it on the street. Commitment to a state hospital with a diagnosis of ambulatory schizophrenia was recommended.

Discussion. This case also illustrates the relationship between breaking and entering, voyeurism, and fantasies of possession of a female. A fantasy of acceptance by a female is combined with the fantasy of subduing and neutralizing a dangerously overpowering object. His sadistic daydreams are in direct relationship with feeling of impotence, weakness, and inferiority. This case illustrates the insufficiency of the legal machinery for public protection.

Case 3

An 18-year-old boy drove a 15-year-old girl acquaintance to an isolated place where he tore off her clothes, strangled her with a plastic belt, stuffed her mouth with tissue paper, and then dragged her body into the bushes. Following the murder, he attended the afternoon session in school and the same evening he drove to New York to attend a Billy Graham rally. The shocked neighbors described the boy as "a nice quiet kid" and "too deeply religious to go out with girls." What the neighbors did not know was that at the age of 14 years he had been an in-patient at the Diagnostic Center for the following reasons. He forced two little girls to undress and then stuffed tissue paper into their mouths; he broke into a neighbor's house, ripped woman's clothes and strewed paper, coffee and sugar through the house. Prior to the incident he was angered by his parents and he felt that the lady of the house into which he broke, was contemptuous of him.

Projective tests revealed hostility to women, fear of inadequacy and competition. The mother was described as overprotective and rejecting at the same time. I re-examined and checked him while he was in the state prison for several months. At the initial interview, he claimed amnesia for the events but then he revealed the incident in the form of a dream. He said that he dreamt he picked up the girl on the way to school and since it was early he was just riding around. In the car, she made some kind of a motion towards him and she started to play with the zipper on her skirt. He took her to an isolated place and he was going to rip off her clothes, but at this point he woke up.

In the subsequent interviews, he described his dismay, anxiety and disappointment evoked by the victim's seductive behavior with boys.

He was preoccupied with the moral aspects of her flirtatiousness and, when she started playing with her zipper while riding in his car, he became anxious, excited, and angry because "she disappointed me". After the murder, he was relieved. For several days prior to the discovery of the body, he did not feel as if he had committed the crime. On one occasion, I saw him drawing a space ship which he intended to send to Washington, D.C. in order "to do something for the country." When asked whether the space ship would work, he answered after some reflection that perhaps his ideas were foolish. He frequently smiled inappropriately and was emotionally flat.

DISCUSSION. This case has the earmarks of compulsive repetitiveness, as well as a catathymic reaction with discharge of tension. Previous attacks on little girls, a bizarre episode of breaking and entering with destruction of female clothing, sexual inhibition and preoccupation with sexual morality, form the basic picture.

Case 4

A 22-year-old young man killed his girlfriend with multiple stabs during an automobile ride. Since her father forbade her to see him, he waited in his parked car on her way to work. The incident was described by him as an ego-alien and dream-like experience. While stabbing her, he also kissed her, and when she fell dead on the floor his first impression was that she just joked. While driving around with the dead body, he had a vague thought of suicide. He then loaded his gun, drove to an isolated place, shot the ammunition, and surrendered to the state police with a note, "Gladys and I sinned."

The murder was preceded by several months of vague homicidal and suicidal fantasies. Several weeks prior to the event he borrowed a knife, sharpened it, and told a friend he was going to kill the girl. Although these thoughts seemed to him as unreal, he was afraid to see her alone for three weeks prior to the incident. He cried in church because of these preoccupations and he approached his pastor, his father, and his friend but no one understood his plight and nothing was done to relieve him. Shortly afterwards, he drove with a loaded gun to his girlfriend's house. The scenery on the way seemed to him to be unreal. Suddenly, a thought of throwing the gun away occurred to him and he returned home. He described this experience as follows: "Holy cow. What am I doing here? It was like a dream." The day of the murder he had a gun and a sharpened knife in his car. Yet, he was angered by the suggestion of premeditation and planning. He said, “They all think that I planned it. It was just in my mind. I never thought it would happen. I never really meant it.”

He felt relieved after his arrest since, “I do not have to worry about her any more.” In jail he had fantasies and daydreams of throwing the girlfriend off a cliff, shooting her, having a snake bite her, and so forth. At one of the interviews, he said that he felt it was right to kill her, giving this explanation: “It is kind of funny . . . when I asked the Lord for guidance, I thought of Abraham making a sacrifice of Isaac . . . by killing her and myself, the sins would be washed away. We had been sinning for having sex . . . sex mostly.” He then recited allegedly from the Bible: “To be carnally minded is death . . . to be spiritually minded is peace and joy.”

The defendant was raised in a large family with a somewhat aggressive mother and religiously preoccupied father. He left school in his freshman year. He was discharged from the Armed Forces after six months of service, most of it spent in an Army hospital with complaints of backache. His work record was unimpressive and he was idle most of the time. With strangers, he was shy and felt inferior. He shied away from the opposite sex. He used to hit his little sister and inflict pain on other girls in close contact with him. Only after a few months of courtship, he mistreated and abused his girlfriend physically.

DISCUSSION. This case illustrates a progressive buildup of tension derived from obsessive preoccupations with sexual morality, eventually leading to the elimination of the source of conflict through murder. The fantasies of homicide preceding the murder were perceived as ego-alien rather than as conscious planning. In the struggle with the growing impulse to kill, his call for help remained unheeded. An element of minor sadism toward females was elicited in the background history. Yet, a definite source of conflict inducing an unbearable psychological situation was necessary for the final explosion.

REFERENCES

1. Guttmacher, M. S. (1951). *Sex offenses – The problem, causes and prevention.* New York: W. W. Norton and Co.
2. Hirschfield, M. (1944). *Sexual anomalies and perversions.* London: Francis Aldor.
3. Krafft-Ebing. (1934). *Psychopathia sexualis* –transl. New York: F. J. Rebman, Physicians and Surgeons Book Co.

4. De River, P. (1949). *The sexual criminal.* Springfield, IL: Charles C Thomas.
5. Karpman, B. (1954). *The sexual offender and his offenses.* New York: Julian Press Inc.
6. Wilson, C. & Pitman, P. (1962). *Encyclopedia of murder.* New York: Putnam and Sons.
7. Revitch, E. (1957). Sex Murder and Sex Aggression. *J. Med. Soc. N.J., 54*: 519-524.
8. Lerner, M. *New York Post,* Apr. 22, 1957.
9. Brancale, R., Ellis, A., Doorbar, R. (1952). Psychiatric and psychological investigations of convicted sex offenders. *Am. J. of Psychiat, 109*: 17-21.
10. Brancale, R., Vuocolo, A., Mc Neil D. (1965). Diagnostic Center report, *Welfare Reporter, 16*:3-9.
11. Revitch, E. & Weiss, R. (1962). The pedophiliac offender. *Dis. Nerv. Syst., 23*:73-78.
12. Wertham, F. (1937). The catathymic crisis. *Arch. Neurol. & Psychiat., 37*: 974-977.
13. Hill, P. (1960). *Portrait of a sadist.* New York: Avon Book Division.
14. Guttmacher, M. (1963). Dangerous offenders. *Crime and delinquency, 9*:381-390.
15. Kennedy, F., Hoffman, H. R., & Haines, W. (1947). Psychiatric study of William Heirens. *J. of Crim. Law and Criminology, 38*:311-341.
16. Freeman, L. (1956). *Catch me before I kill more.* New York: Pocket Books.
17. Brancale, R. (1960). Personal Communication.
18. Deshais, G. (1954). Les reactions anti-sociales dans la mayenne-ann. *Med. Psychol, 112*:192-211.
19. Wertham, F. (1950). *Dark legend.* New York: Doubleday Co.
20. Woddis, G. M. (1957). Depression and crime. *Brit. J. of Delinquency, 8*:85-94.
21. Easson, W. M., & Steinhilber, R. M. (1961). Murderous aggression in children and adolescents. *Arch. Gen. Psychiat., 4*:1-9.
22. Berkowitz, L. (1963). *Aggressive stimuli, aggressive responses and hostility catharsis in violence and war.* Edited by J. Masserman. New York: Grune and Stratton.
23. Satten, J., Menninger, K., Rosen, I. & Mayman, M. (1960). Murder without apparent motive. *Am. J. Psychiat., 117*:48-53.
24. Williams, A. H. (1964). The psychopathology and treatment of sexual murderers. Edited by I. Rosen. In *The pathology and treatment of sexual deviation.* New York: Oxford Univ. Press.
25. Wertham, F. (1949). *The show of violence.* New York: Eton Brooks, Inc.

Chapter 4

GYNOCIDE AND UNPROVOKED ATTACKS ON WOMEN

The purpose of this paper is to present the phenomenology, diagnosis, dynamics, and prognosis of sexually motivated attacks on, and murder of, women by males. The underlying sexual pathology of these attacks is not always recognized. The legal profession may look, in some cases, for "logical" reasons such as robbery or jealousy, while the offender himself may not be able to offer an explanation, or he too may evoke a "logical" motivation. As far as I know, there are no available statistical data of sexually motivated murders and assaults. The extrapolation from press releases and from the newspaper reports of the current Florida trial of Theodore R. Bundy,[1] who is suspected of murdering 18 to 36 women in four states within a period of four years, suggests about 50 to 75 such murders and an unknown number of attacks a year in the United States. Whatever the incidence may be, the number is negligible in comparison with the frequency of sexual offenses and other types of murder. In popular fantasy, the sex offender is an aggressive and dangerous rapist and killer. The studies by Brancale et al.[2,3] indicate that the majority of sex offenders referred by the court to the New Jersey State Diagnostic Center, under the purview of the New Jersey Sex Offender Law,[4] were passive, inadequate, non-aggressive individuals. Out of the initial 1,206 sex offenders referred to the Diagnostic Center, only 110 used force. Most of the sex offenses were non-violent and non-coital.

Source: Revitch, E. (1980). Gynocide and unprovoked attacks on women. *Correctional and Social Psychiatry, 26*:6-11.

PHENOMENOLOGY

Sexually motivated murders of males by males are less frequent than murders of females by males. The most recent case is that of John Gacy. Male bodies with evidence of torture were found buried under his home. Haarman and Denke in post World War I Germany enticed young men to their homes, where the victims were butchered and their flesh prepared for sale.[5] Woman may also entertain sadistic fantasies and kill. Magnus Hirshfeld[6] described a female patient who fantasied killing women and drinking their blood. This improved with psychotherapy. Elizabeth Brownrigg in seventeeth century England sadistically mistreated her servant girls. This resulted in death of one of the girls which lead to Brownrigg's execution.[5]

Some of the male attackers and killers of women may also victimize men, children, and animals. The most striking example is that of Peter Kurten in post World War I Germany. Kurten stabbed sheep while violating them sexually; he choked and mistreated women while courting them; he sadistically murdered and mutilated women, men and children; on one occasion he killed a swan and drank its blood.[5] Some of these murders may be associated with necrophilia,[7] vampirism (drinking of blood), cannibalism, and mutilation of the body.[6,8] A strange case of cannibalism was reported by Wertham in the case of Albert Fish.[9] Fish abducted a 10-year-old girl and, after killing her, he cooked her flesh and ate it with great excitement.

The killing of children by pedophiles is rare, since most pedophiliac offenses are of a noncoital and non-aggressive nature.[10] The most striking case is that of the French nobleman Gilles de Rais in the fithteenth century. After the end of the Hundred Year War, in which Rais fought the English under Joan of Arc, he withdrew into one of his castles. With the help of his underlings, he kidnapped, tortured sexually, molested, and killed about 150 peasant children of both sexes living in his domain. It was disclosed at his trial that he kissed the severed heads and, in the presence of his accomplices, he sexually violated the victims' bodies. Such extreme cases, however, are rare, although the enormity of the perversion makes the press and is recorded in the annals of crime.

Most commonly the victims are battered, choked or knifed, with or without manifestations of sexuality, such as rape or attempted rape, erection and ejaculation.[12,13] Some cases of attacks on women are associated with breaking and entering. The act of burglary itself may be sexually motivated. Voyeurism impulses, transvestism, stealing of female undergarments, ripping female clothes, masturbatory fantasies of breaking into homes, and overt sexual excitement in entering the premises are characteristic in these types of burglars. The attacks on women may occur during or independently of breaking and entering. The following two cases previously reported[13,14] will be extracted for illustration.

Case 1

A 17-year-old youth was referred for psychiatric evaluation as a result of following an adolescent girl on the street and hitting her without provocation with a stick. This was preceded by an argument with his sister. His motive, as he said, was hatred "for the whole female race." At the age of 21 years, I re-examined him because of indecent communications to females, touching sales girls in stores, and voyeuristic acts. At the age of 24 years, four months after his release from prison, he broke into a house through a window and hit a sleeping young woman on the head with a lead pipe. He was unimpressive looking, weakly-built with a stooped posture. He disclosed fantasies of being a S.S. officer in a concentration camp, "burning people in ovens" or a conqueror killing female hostages.

Case 2

A 19-year-old soldier, whom I examined on the prison ward of a station hospital during World War II, used to break into homes since the age of 12 years in order to hit sleeping women with a brick. These acts relieved him of inner tension and depression.

Mistreatment and killing of cats may have a particular significance. The most striking example is a man 42 years old, at the time I examined him, who had served prison sentences half of his lifetime for repeated burglaries. On one occasion, he followed a woman and hit her on the head with a stick for no obvious reason. He also experienced a feeling of triumph when he mistreated, killed, and burned cats whom he compared with women.[14] Many of these individuals entertain sadistic fantasies which may precede assaults by years. One of my cases attacked a woman in order to tie her legs after fantasing such an occurrence for 31 years.[12] The aggressive fantasies may be discovered accidentally. The following case is abstracted from a previous publication.[12]

Case 3

A 35-year-old man serving a sentence for larceny was referred for a psychiatric evaluation by the prison authorities. The custodial officers, in checking his cell, found pictures he had drawn of the torture of women in medieval dungeons, and hundreds of pages of horror stories of torture he had composed while in confinement. There was no history of aggressive behavior.

The following case illustrates the depression and inner torture accompanying sadistic fantasies which, eventually may end, not in assault, but in suicide.

Case 4

A 23-year-old man had been referred for psychiatric evaluation because he was disturbed by an erection while killing an opossum with a spear. He had a long history of killing small animals by breaking their necks. In the interview, he was in excellent contact, coherent, expressing his concern freely and relevantly. In spite of this, he lacked warmth and seemed to be distant. He revealed a lifelong preoccupation with violence and he even mentioned that under Hitler he would probably have killed people. He also fantasied about being a Gestapo officer. In his masturbatory fantasies, he raped women. He had difficulties in dating girls because of a fear of harming them. The motive of power was dominant in his account. He also entertained strange suicidal fantasies such as having his hands cut off by an electric saw so that he would die of exsanguination. The significant facts of his background history were his mother's two divorces and a third marriage, and his perception of his mother as seductive and promiscuous. After about two years of psychotherapy with a psychologist, his sadistic fantasies weakened, and he even shared an apartment with a young woman. He committed suicide when he seemed to be improving.

DIAGNOSIS AND CLASSIFICATION

Out of the 43 initial cases of assaults on and murder of women and men, 19 were considered to be schizoid, nine clinically schizophrenic, five mentally defective, and 10 had personality disorders.[13] The psychiatric diagnosis per se, however, most of the time does not explain the criminal act and is inadequate for the classification of offenders. The common denominator in criminal activities are the motivational stimuli leading to the offense. The motivational stimuli are spectrally distributed with the chiefly exogenous stimuli on one, and the chiefly endogenously derived stimuli on the other end of the spectrum. The scale is thus divided into (1) environmentally stimulated crimes, (2) situational crimes, (3) impulsive crimes, (4) catathymic crimes, and (5) compulsive crimes.[15,16] Transitional forms are common, since no human behavior can be tightly fit into a rigid category. Most of the sexually motivated assaults and murders belong to the compulsive, and some to the catathymic group. The beatings by impulsive individuals, the attacks and murders of women during robbery, mugging or quarrels, most of the time have no underlying sexual significance and, therefore, will not be discussed in this paper.

COMPULSIVE ATTACKS AND MURDERS

In these cases, the need to commit the act is compelling and with a strong potential for repetition. They should not be confused with the obsessive-compulsive neurotics except for the compelling character of the act. Some of these offenders attempt to resist the need, and this usually brings on severe anxiety with somatic manifestations. Krafft-Ebing[8] reported and described a 20-year-old man who attacked and stabbed girls in the genitals in broad daylight: "For a while he succeeded in mastering his morbid craving, but this produced feelings of anxiety and a copious perspiration would break out from his entire body." William Heirens, whose career of killing women started with repetitive burglaries and stealing female undergarments, had headaches and sweating when he resisted his compulsion.[17] A 16-year-old boy with a history of burglaries, vandalism, and murder of two women in their homes, struggled against his compulsion by praying at bedtime not to wake up in the morning so that he would not have to commit crimes.[18]

The attacks and murders may be committed in a similar ritualistic manner, but this is not always the case. They may be frequent or isolated and repeated at long intervals. The compulsion may persist and continue after years of imprisonment. The following two cases are illustrative:

Case 5

A 23-year-old ex-marine killed and mutilated a 15-year-old girl. The victim's skull was crushed, the right breast showed traces of biting, the left eye was destroyed, and both jaws were fractured. The offender was sentenced to the electric chair and he spent close to 15 years in the death house. His sentence was eventually commuted. While on parole, he abducted a woman and wounded her with a knife while she was trying to escape from his car. Several interviews in the death house revealed an asocial, psychopathic-like, but not criminal pattern of behavior. In adolescence, however, he had been placed on probation for attacking a girl, throwing her to the ground, and exhibiting himself to her. He was of high intelligence, sensitive, without a thinking disorder, but guarded and defensive. He denied his guilt until he was apprehended following the knife attack.

Case 6

A 46-year-old man with fetishism of leather gloves and purses worn by women had been sentenced to life for the murder of a woman. The murder occurred while he was under psychiatric care for his fetishism, burglaries, and assaults on women. In prison, he was a model inmate, and even obtained a master's degree while confined. After 14 years of imprisonment, he was re-arrested after only four days on parole for assaulting seven women with a pipe and grabbing their leather purses. He was suspected of other murders of women in the surrounding communities.

The following case is illustrative of a compulsive strangler:

Case 7

A 26-year-old window cleaner was referred for psychiatric examination as he was a suspect in strangling to death a mother and her married daughter. Suspicion was aroused because he worked in the house a day before the two women were found dead, and because he was arrested for strangling (but not killing) an elderly woman. The prosecutor doubted the suspect's guilt because of negative polygraph findings and because a hypnotist, called in on the case, believed he was not guilty of murder. Furthermore, suicide was suspected because both victims were found hanging. The suspect had a history of threatening and raping his friend's girlfriend in her apartment, and of choking, but not killing, an elderly woman in the same apartment house. In adolescence, he choked his sister and struck his mother. He had a prison sentence for hitting a man with a bat during an argument and, in his youth, he was considered to be a juvenile delinquent. He was raised in a culturally and economically deprived and emotionally disturbed family. In the interview, he was friendly but dull. At first he denied guilt, but under sodium amobarbital injected intravenously, he spoke of a "sex fanatic" who had killed the women, giving a detailed description of the "sex fanatic" who had committed the offense. Once in state prison, he sent me a letter admitting to his guilt and describing the details of the offense.

CATATHYMIC MURDERS AND ASSAULTS

The concept of catathymic crisis was introduced into psychiatric criminology by Wertham.[19] In essence, a catathymic crisis is a release of accumulated psychic tension through an exploding aggression. The aggression is due to a threat to the intrapsychic homeostasis. The dynamic factors responsible for this threat, in our cases, are an intensification of sexual inadequacy and of incestuous or homosexual conflicts during a short or prolonged ambivalent relationship with a woman. Sudden murder of women by men, either during a brief contact or after a prolonged relationship, are the most common catathymic homicides. The catathymic murder during a prolonged relationship is characterized by three stages: induction, aggressive act, and relief. The induction stage may last close to a year or perhaps longer. Here, the perpetrator is preoccupied with suicidal, a mixture of suicidal and homicidal, or only homicidal fantasies directed against his female companion. Behavior may become bizarre and schizophrenic-like. The mood is depressed. The subject may warn friends, his minister, or his psychiatrist of his intent, but no attention is usually paid to his warnings.

The *Tarasoff* case in California was very likely a catathymic murder. The perpetrator warned his psychiatrist of his intent, apparently pleading for help, but police did not detain him since he "looked normal." A similar case recently occurred in New Jersey, where the treating psychiatrist failed to notify either the police or the girl's family, which lead to a lawsuit against the doctor.

Case 8

The following case was reported previously[13] and will be summarized as an illustration of a catathymic murder. A 22-year-old man killed his girlfriend with multiple stab wounds and then surrendered to the state police. During the approximately 9 months of courtship, he developed suicidal and homicidal ideas directed against his girlfriend. On one occasion, he drove her home with a loaded rifle, but he threw the weapon away. He warned his friends and his minister of his intent, but no attention was paid to his plea, except that the minister prayed with him. When I examined him in prison, he quoted the Bible and he said that killing the girl, and his own planned suicide, would wash away the sin of having had sexual relations with her. Later, the homicidal and suicidal fantasies were perceived as ego-alien rather than conscious planning. He said, "They all think that I planned it. It was just in my mind. I never thought it would happen."

Case 9

I first examined this person at the New Jersey State Diagnostic Center and followed him as an in-patient when he was 14 years old for running away from home on numerous occasions and for an episode of breaking and entering. He was of high intelligence, pleasant, and cooperative with the staff. A sad history of abandonment by a sexually promiscuous and alcoholic mother, and indifference and hostility by his father and stepmother, was elicited.

Interviews and the projective tests revealed confused sexual identity, feelings of inadequacy, resentment of his mother, and perception of sex as dangerous, "awful" and "dirty." Three years later, he attempted suicide and was committed to a state hospital. Fourteen years after the first examination, I received a letter from an attorney in another state with the following information: The patient, now 28 years old was married, father of children and employed in cleaning, repair, and maintenance jobs by a cleaning company. The day of the incident he was doing his work while the lady of the house was working at her sewing machine. He told her, with some concern, that her baby was screaming upstairs, but she did not seem to pay attention to it. Then, for no obvious reason, he pulled a handgun from his waistband, grabbed her around the waist, threw her on the floor and kneeled straddling her legs. She pleaded not to hurt her, promising to cooperate, but he tied her hands and mouth in order not to hear her screaming. He then pulled her slacks off, turned her around and shot her with two bullets. He remembered being fascinated by the sound of blood spilling on the floor. After the murder, he felt horrified, left the cleaning gear in the house and left. He spent the night with friends who notified the police of the incident. The victim's seeming indifference to her baby's screams, and her promise to cooperate, very likely unleashed the negative emotions to his rejecting and promiscuous mother.

PSYCHOPATHOLOGY

Hostility to women, preoccupation with maternal sexual conduct, overt or covert incestuous preoccupations, feelings of sexual inferiority, weakness, and inadequacy, and occasionally, a need to completely possess and own the victim, are the most common findings in the thought content of these offenders. In the background, there is either maternal overprotection, infantilization and seduction, or outright rejection of the son. Maternal sexual indiscretions real or fantasized are also common. I examined an 11-year-old boy for several attempts to choke little girls. Under sodium amobarbital injected intravenously, he revealed witnessing mother's sexual relations with various men. The boy was sexually preoccupied and he made profane remarks about his mother's activities. Choking girls, he said, made him feel "glad." Another 14-year-old boy was examined for beating, choking and stabbing a 10-year-old girl. He expressed dislike for all the girls and he revealed a fantasy of his mother's purity and absence of sexual relations between his parents.

I gained a surprising insight into murder of women during psychotherapy with a 55-year-old professional. He had been in treatment with various psychiatrists for half of his lifetime. In addition to vague homosexual fantasies, and a feeling of victimization by his superiors in the company, he also had serious marital problems punctuated by occasional violence. In connection with these difficulties, he said after several years of psychotherapy, "The only way of handling female authority is to try to kill the woman or try to cheapen her and to put her in a bad light." With this statement, he summarized the essential elements in the psychopathology of gynocide. This patient felt that in his youth he had been overprotected and infantilized by his mother.

There is an indication that some of the attacks by predisposed individuals may be unleashed by a suggestive stimulus. Thus, Gilles de Rais, in his own words at his trial, was stimulated by reading *Twelve Caesars* written by the Roman historian Suetonius. Henry Bush choked to death three elderly women after seeing the movie *Psycho.*[20] Robert B. Smith, with a history of homicidal fantasies, killed four women and a three-year-old girl, stimulated by the newspaper reports of the Chicago killing of eight nurses.[21]

Freud mentioned the intimate connection between sex and aggression.[22] MacLean[23] pointed to the interconnection and proximity of the limbic structures connected with feeding and aggression (amygdala), and the structures connected with sexual functions (septum, hippocampus). Furthermore, he pointed to the display of genitals in male squirrel monkeys during a fight as another indication of the interconnection between sex and aggression. The feeding and aggressive functions of the amygdala may be the neuroanatomical substrate of cannibalism associated with some cases of gynocide.

PROGNOSIS

The prognosis depends on the personality organization of the offender in terms of ego strength, inner cohesiveness, ethical standards, empathy, and the place the criminal act occupies on the motivational scale. The catathymic aggressions, in general, have a lesser likelihood to be repeated than the compulsive offenses. Cases 5 and 6 illustrate the repetition of aggressive acts after years of imprisonment. Guttmacher[24] reported the case of a 40-year-old man, who 13 years after release from prison, where he served a sentence for killing and mutilation of a prostitute, was again arrested for attacking another prostitute with a knife. Three years later, after serving an 18-month sentence for the previous incident, he killed and beheaded another prostitute.

It is difficult to draw a personality profile of a potentially gynocidal individual because of the variety of psychiatric diagnoses, intelligence, outer appearance, behavior, and past history. Most of the gynocidal offenders have no history of the usual sex crimes. In the 43 cases previously reported,[13] only three had a history of sex offenses. Twelve had a history of breaking and entering, with and without attacks on the female occupants. Certain traits, however, should alert us in helping to find a perpetrator of attacks, when requested by detectives. These traits are: (1) history of unprovoked attacks on women even if they seem insignificant, (2) breaking and entering committed alone and in bizarre circumstances, (3) fetishism and stealing of female undergarments, (4) expressions of contempt, hatred, and fear of women, (5) violence against animals, particularly cats, (6) violent fantasy life, (7) confusion of sexual identity, (8) emotional shallowness and blurring of reality boundaries, (9) preoccupation with sexual morality, and (10) previous warnings by the suspect that he may kill or commit suicide. Preoccupation with sexual morality was the only possible prognostic sign noted in Case 8.

SUMMARY

The problem of sexually motivated attacks on and murder or women by males was presented. Freud indicated the connection of sex with aggression, and MacLean demonstrated the neuroanatomical substrate of this connection in the limbic system. Minor attacks on women and homicidal fantasies may precede the actual gynocide. The murder may be, and may not be, associated with sexual molestation, erection, and ejaculation. Choking, knifing, and battering are the most common methods of attack. On some occasions, the gynocide is associated with cannibalism, vampirism, and necrophilia. Many of these cases have a tendency to repeat aggression against women even after years of imprisonment. In catathymic murders–which are a result of an ambivalent relationship with a female and leads to the disruption of intrapsychic homeostasis–often has a brighter prognosis as to future offenses. Unresolved incestual conflict, infantilization and overprotection by mother, or outright rejection of the son, hatred of women, and preoccupation with sex and sexual morality, were found in the majority of these offenders.

REFERENCES

1. Bundy Guilty Murders of Two Florida Women. *New York Times*, May 25, 1979.
2. Brancale R., Ellis A., & Doorbar, R. (1952). Psychiatric and psychological investigations of convicted sex offenders. *American Journal of Psychiatry, 102*:17-21.
3. Brancale R., MacNeil, D., & Vuocolo, A. (1965). Profile of the New Jersey sex offender: A statistical study of 1206 male sex offenders. *The Welfare Reporter, 16*:3-9.
4. N.J. Statutes Annotated, 2A – 164-3.
5. Wilson, C., Pitman, P. (1962). *Encyclopedia of murder.* New York: G. P. Putnam Sons.
6. Hirschfeld, M. (1944). *Sexual anomalies*. London: Francis Aldor Publishers.
7. Smith, S. M., & Brown, E. (1978). Necrophilia and lust murder: Report of a case occurrence. *Bulletin of the American Academy of Psychiatry and Law, 6*:259-268.
8. Von Krafft-Ebing, R. (1934). *Psychopathia sexualis.* Translation by F. G.Rebman, (originally published, 1886). New York: Physicians and Surgeons Book Company.
9. Wertham, F. (1949). *The show of violence.* New York: Eton Books Inc.
10. Revitch, E., & Weiss, R. (1962). The pedophiliac offender. *Diseases of the Nervous System, 23*:73-78.
11. Benedetti, Y. (1972). *Gilles de Rais.* New York: Stein and Day Publishers.
12. Revitch, E. (1957). Sex murder and sex aggression. *Journal of The Medical Society of New Jersey, 54*:19-24.
13. Revitch, E. (1965). Sex murder and the potential sex murderer. *Diseases of the Nervous System, 26*:640-648.
14. Revitch, E. (1978). Sexually motivated burglaries. *Bulletin of the American Academy of Psychiatry and the Law, 6*:277-283.
15. Revitch, E. (1975). Psychiatric evaluation and classification of antisocial activities. *Diseases of the Nervous System, 36*:419-421.
16. Revitch, E. (1977). Classification of offenders for prognostic and dispositional evaluation. *Bulletin of the American Academy of Psychiatry and the Law, 15*:41-50.
17. Kennedy, F., Hoffman, M., & Haines, W. (1947). A study of William Heirens. *American Journal of Psychiatry, 104*:113-121.
18. Revitch, E., & Schlesinger, L. B. (1978). Murder: Evaluation, classification and prediction. In I. L. Kutash, S. B. Kutash, & L. B. Schlesinger (Eds.), (1998). *Violence: Perspectives on murder and aggression.* San Francisco: Jossey Bass Publishers.

19. Wertham, F. The catathymic crisis: A clinical entity. (1937). *Archives of Neurology and Psychiatry, 37*:974-977.
20. Purse Snatcher Admits Strangling Three Women. *Newark Star Ledger,* Sept. 7, 1960.
21. Cops Sift Past of Arizona Kid. *Daily News,* Nov. 14, 1966.
22. Freud, S. (1938). Three contributions to the theory of sex. In, *The basic writings of Sigmund Freud.* Translated by A. A. Brill. New York: The Modern Library.
23. MacLean, P. D. (1962). New findings relevant to the evolution of psychosexual functions of the brain. *Journal of Nervous and Mental Disease, 135*:289-301.
24. Guttmacher, M. (1963). Dangerous offenders. *Crime and Delinquency. 9*:381-390.

Chapter 5

SEXUALLY MOTIVATED BURGLARIES

Burglary is defined as the unlawful entry of a structure to commit a felony or theft. The rate of burglaries in the U.S. increased 30 percent between 1972 and 1976. Of the persons arrested for burglary in 1976, one-third were juveniles.[1] Although I believe that most crime is stimulated by social environmental causes,[2,3] it is important to recognize that some crimes, including burglary, have a compulsive, symbolic character with overt or covert sexual motivation.

Guttmacher[4] felt that burglary, assault, and cutting cases often have a sexual origin, and he wrote that the burglar's basic personality structure "resembled that of the rapist far more closely than that of the exhibitionist. In fact, the legal term breaking and entering bears such a connotation" (p. 383). Banay[5] also remarked that there "are burglars who tell of achieving orgasm at the moment of entering a window or breaking a locked door" (p. 94). The initial studies by Brancale and others, of the cases referred to the New Jersey State Diagnostic Center under the purview of the New Jersey Sex Offenders Law, clearly indicate that the bulk of sex offenders are basically innocuous, passive, immature individuals committing non-violent and non-coital offenses.[6,7] Only 5 percent were referred for sexual assaults. I found that in 43 cases of serious attacks on women, including beating, choking, knifing, and nine murders, only three offenders had a record of previous sex offenses; 12 had a record of breaking and entering. Four out of the 12 combined breaking and entering with assaults on or threats to the female occupant.[8]

Source: Revitch, E. (1978). Sexually motivated burglaries. *Bulletin of the American Academy of Psychiatry and Law, 6*:277-283.

In my experience, breaking and entering committed alone and under bizarre circumstances, stealing of female underwear, destruction of female clothing, and torture or killing of cats have ominous significance.[8] The well-known case of William Heirens[9,10] is illustrative. At age 17, Heirens entered a house through the window, removed a six-year-old from her bed and cut her body into several pieces. Prior to this, he killed two women in their homes. His career of murders was preceded by burglaries which started at the age of nine years. Initially he stole female underwear. A few years later, he experienced sexual excitement, with erection and occasional ejaculation, while breaking into homes through windows. These acts were accompanied by a state of depersonalization. On many occasions, Heirens tried to resist his compulsion, but this effort resulted in headaches, sweats, and tearing the sheets off his bed.[10,11] Krafft-Ebing[12] described a patient's similar feeling of anxiety, with copious perspiration, when he attempted to control his compulsion to slap, pinch, or cut the genitals of women.

I have previously reported three cases of attacks on women along with breaking and entering.[3,8] One individual burglarized a home and ripped female clothes at the age of 13, and at the age of 19 he strangled a 15-year-old girl. The second offender, with a history of voyeurism and sadistic fantasies directed against women, broke into a house through the window and hit the sleeping female occupant with a pipe. The third individual, a 37-year-old man, broke into several dwellings and choked and raped the elderly occupants; he did this within a month of his release from serving a prison sentence for burglaries. His history was replete with violence and sadistic acts against animals.

Unfortunately, we do not have data on the relative frequency with which burglaries are sexually motivated. My impression is that the phenomenon is not uncommon. Some cases taken from my files over the years will illustrate the problem. Because most of the cases were collected at the New Jersey State Diagnostic Center, there is a disproportionately large number of juveniles, since juvenile offenders were more likely to be referred for inpatient evaluation than adult offenders. Many offenders provide logical explanations for their offenses; however, the "logical" act such as larceny or robbery is only a cover-up for bizarre and frequently obscure impulses. This is illustrated in my report of a 40-year-old man, without a previous criminal history, who served a sentence for attempted robbery. His offense, however, was stimulated by a longstanding compulsion to tie women's legs.[13]

CASE REPORTS

Case 1

A 19-year-old soldier was examined on the prison ward of an army station hospital during World War II, following an arrest for breaking and entering and assault on a sleeping occupant of the house. In the interview, he was neat and cooperative, describing his life history and the present incident in great detail. He described a life of deprivation, poverty, and poor school and work adjustment. In the army, however, he performed to the satisfaction of his superiors. He reported that since age 12 he had had an urge to enter homes and to hit the female occupant while she was asleep. The woman's screams and fright gave him a feeling of triumph and dispelled his feeling of dejection.

He described the most recent incident as follows. He felt an urge to enter a home earlier in the day. For this purpose, he obtained a pass to town. After drinking beer with another soldier and having intercourse with a pick-up, he walked through the town. At 2:00 a.m. he noticed a house with the front door open, so that he could see the light reflecting into a polished hallway floor. He told his friend to wait and he entered the house with a brick and a piece of rock he had picked up earlier on the street. "I entered the room and saw a woman sleeping. I then just went over to her and hit her head with the brick. She started screaming. I dropped the brick and ran down the hall and out. I do not know just why I hit this woman. I guess I could not help myself. I've always had a desire to hit somebody. I would also hurt my brothers and sisters. When I feel sad or blue, and I hit somebody and hurt them and make them scream, it makes me feel happy again."

Case 2

A 16-year-old boy was referred for psychiatric evaluation on charges of breaking and entering, run-away, and sniffing gasoline. According to his mother, he was verbally and psychically abusive, destructive, and uncontrollable. He was hostile and belligerent upon admission to the ward. In two interviews under the influence of intravenously injected amobarbital sodium, he revealed a series of voyeuristic incidents hoping to see a woman in the process of undressing. At home he masturbated, revisualizing the women he spied upon. Only one episode of breaking and entering was known to the court. In the interviews, he reported several additional incidents. The first incident took place in the evening. When he saw a house with an open window, he suddenly had an impulse to "look around" and inspect the interior of the dwelling. He entered through the open window and inspected the living room, bedroom, and kitchen. He took 35 cents out of a pile of a few dollars and left. The seven burglaries he reported took place under similar circumstances and only in the last few incidents did he take a few dollars upon leaving.

Case 3

A 16-year-old boy was referred by the juvenile court because he was found at night on the street wearing female clothes. He had appeared previously in court on charges of breaking, entering, and larceny. While in the dwelling, he attired himself in female clothing and masturbated. Upon admission to the ward he was withdrawn and uninvolved. In the interviews, he admitted to four incidents of breaking and entering for the purpose of stealing female clothing. He used the clothes for masturbation in the bedrooms of the homes he entered. While masturbating, he visualized himself as being a girl. On the projective tests, aggressive feelings and death wishes toward parents were elicited.

Case 4

A 16-year-old boy was referred for inpatient study by the juvenile court on a technical charge of incorrigibility. He had been treated previously in a psychiatric clinic where he was described as isolated, withdrawn, hostile, with unrealistic thinking, and with a tendency to transvestism. He had been a premature infant and had to repeat kindergarten and first grade. His family history was replete with epilepsy and mental illness. Since early life, he had handled and ripped female clothes. The projective tests pointed to isolation, poor self-image, poor reality testing, and female identification. In the interviews, he reported an urge to masturbate while wearing female apparel and to "think crazy thoughts." After some prodding, he revealed masturbatory fantasies of breaking into stores through a window, of seeing his mother naked, and of looking through a window with a telescope and seeing couples engaged in intercourse. On one occasion, unknown to the court, he actually entered a store through the window, and he became sexually aroused. He wanted to masturbate, but he was too frightened to complete the act.

Case 5

A 12-year-old boy was referred for inpatient evaluation by the juvenile court because of repeated breaking and entering. In several homes, he had stolen money, beer, or food. In others, he had left without taking anything. On the ward, he was unpopular with his peer group. He was big for his age, overweight, with small genitals, so that the diagnosis of Frohlich's Syndrome was considered. He was exceedingly preoccupied with sex. He drew a penis over the door of a boy's room; he approached other boys with an offer to commit sodomy; and he bragged about having sexual relations with girls. He treated smaller and weaker boys sadistically and forced one of them to suck his nipple. In the interviews, he was evasive and lacked spontaneity. He revealed, however, a dream of entering a store and opening the cash register. He admitted to entering a home through an open door, looking around, opening drawers, and inspecting their contents. He felt proud of this exploit. In two interviews, under the influence of intravenously injected amobarbital sodium and methedrine, he was spontaneous and talkative. He spoke about being sexually aroused by seeing his mother naked in the bathtub and said that while breaking into homes he fantasized about seeing a naked woman. On one occasion, he actually saw a woman sleeping in the house, and he had an urge to lift her skirt, but he was too fearful. Nine years later, I contacted his parents and learned that he was then serving a three-to-six-year sentence for burglary.

Case 6

A 42-year-old male was examined in the state prison and then referred by the authorities to the Diagnostic Center for further evaluation and possible therapy. He had spent at least 20 of his 42 years in various penal institutions throughout the United States, serving sentences for breaking and entering. The current imprisonment had been a consequence of burglaries committed within one month following the completion of an eight-year sentence in a Midwest prison. I saw him in three interviews in six weeks. The third interview was conducted under superficial stages of hypnosis. Following the third session, he claimed to be relieved because he could talk to someone and be understood. Although he left the office, he returned while I was out and escaped through the window with my coat and gloves. When apprehended by the guards he cried and looked pitiful.

In the interviews, he wept while reminiscing about his past and gave an appearance of seeking psychiatric help for its own sake rather than for secondary gain. He said that he started stealing at the age of 11 years. He described a deprived childhood and rejection by his mother. He indicated feeling of inferiority, inner tension, and multiple somatic complaints. On many occasions, he stole instead of keeping a date with a girl. With stolen money, he treated people in bars thus feeling important and admired. He described himself as very sentimental and said that he wept at a movie when "they showed an orphanage with little children and a movie actress giving them toys."

Under hypnosis he revealed killing cats and then burning them. Then he added, "A cat is dainty like a woman. It keeps itself clean, washes itself. It is small. A cat has a woman's face. In fact, you can associate a woman with the cat family by their features. Cats, they are slinky like women. During sexual intercourse I never tried to hit a woman or bruise her." In another interview, he said, "When I set fires or killed cats I had the same feeling as when I entered homes and took jewels or hundreds of dollars." He freely associated and said, "Once I followed a woman and hit her with a stick and then I ran away. I did not want to rape her." He could not explain the reason for this sudden and unprovoked act. He expressed a great deal of resentment against his mother and added that he had begun killing cats when he felt particularly rejected by her.

Case 7

A 35-year-old married man was referred for psychiatric evaluation after convictions on one charge of breaking and entering with intent to commit assault and battery and two charges of lewdness (exhibitionistic acts). He was a college graduate who occupied a good position in industry. Six years prior to the charges he had been on probation for making indecent phone calls. Two years later he had started exhibiting himself to females, and on many occasions he masturbated during the act. The two last exhibitionistic episodes had occurred under the following circumstances. He had a strong urge to exhibit himself when he noticed a woman stopping the car in front of her house. Since the door was not locked, he entered the premises with his genitals exhibited. When the woman screamed, he covered her mouth with his hand and made threatening gestures with a knife he carried with him. A few days later he called the victim on the phone and apologized. A month later he had another urge to exhibit himself. This time he stopped his car, picked out one of the dwellings and knocked at the door. He left when the lady of the house appeared and saw him with his genitals exposed.

The projective tests indicated confused sexual identification, hostility and aggression toward women, and an underlying homosexual component. In the face-to-face interview, and in the interview conducted under the influence of intravenous amobarbital sodium and methedrine, he revealed a poor relationship with his wife and such closeness to his mother that he visited her at least four evenings a week. He also admitted to having had passing homosexual fantasies.

He rationalized his carrying a knife by saying that he needed it to protect his wife in case someone might attack her. The exhibitionistic acts were accompanied by a feeling of triumph, but as soon as the act was over he felt guilty and depressed. When he entered the home with his genitals exhibited and threatened the woman with his knife, he experienced a triumphant feeling off having proved himself. He expressed voyeuristic fantasies during his indecent phone calls by asking the female victims whether they had sexual relations with their boyfriends or with other men. During the calls, he fantasized and masturbated.

COMMENT

The seven cases presented here were chosen to illustrate the various features of sexually motivated burglaries. Some of these burglaries may impress the court or other observers as offenses committed for gain, particularly if valuables had been stolen and no female occupants had been sexually molested. However, the psychiatric evaluation, bolstered by projective tests, may disclose the symbolic nature of the act. Voyeuristic impulses during breaking and entering among burglars seem to be quite common (Cases 2, 4, 5, 7). This may be expressed as an urge to look around, to inspect open drawers, to see a naked woman, or in various voyeuristic fantasies. Overt sexual excitement upon illicitly entering a house was illustrated in the case of William Heirens and also in Case 4. Masturbatory fantasies of breaking into a house, in some cases, further illustrates the sexual symbolism of the act.

Transvestism, stealing of female underwear, or ripping of female clothes are sometimes encountered in juvenile burglars and may be of ominous significance. The case of William Heirens is an illustration, but objective statistical data of such a connection are not available. In addition to covert, symbolic expression in sexually motivated burglaries, there are also openly expressed aggressive acts against females connected with the illicit entering. These acts are accompanied by a feeling of revenge and triumph. The offender in Case 7 experienced triumphal feelings when he exhibited himself to unsuspecting females, and particularly when he entered the house with his genitals exposed and threatened the female occupant with a knife. Exhibitionists, however, are generally innocuous and nonaggressive. I have seen only one other exception, in a case of a man who threw women down to the ground and experienced a feeling of triumph while exhibiting himself. During the exhibitionistic act, most experience a fantasy of being admired by the victim, and a feeling that the act will result in closeness to the victim, who will eventually exhibit her own genitals.

The individual in Case 6 deserves a special mention, for it illustrates the connection between seemingly gain-oriented repetitive burglaries and covert sexual motivation. This patient equated the emotions experienced while breaking into homes with triumphal feelings he experienced in killing cats. In light hypnosis, he compared cats with women and spontaneously stated that he had started killing cats after experiencing severe rejection by his mother, and that on one occasion he had followed a woman and hit her with a stick for no obvious reason. It takes little imagination to follow the sequence of breaking into homes, resentment of mother, killing cats, and hitting a woman. The possibility of dangerous attacks on women by sexually motivated burglars, is suggested by the fact that some have an overt sadistic component and hatred of women similar to that elicited in cases of lust murder.

Elsewhere I have expressed my view[8] that "unprovoked assaults on women, particularly choking and stabbing; offenses of breaking and entering committed solo and in bizarre circumstances; fetishism of underclothing; expression of hatred, contempt or fear of women; violence against animals particularly violence against cats; violent and primitive fantasy life; confusion of sexual identity" may presage a murderous attack on women. By this, I do not mean to imply that any sexually motivated burglar will kill or seriously assault a woman, but in cases of bizarre murders of females, compulsive burglars with a history of minor attacks on women should be investigated by the police.

Only isolated cases can be followed by one examiner, and this material is not sufficient for a comprehensive statistical analysis. Issues of criminal responsibility are irrelevant for prevention because in the majority of these cases, albeit sometimes dangerous and always disturbed, these offenders do not fall under the legal definition of insanity.

SUMMARY

Overt or covert sexual motivation was found in several repetitive, compulsive burglars. Voyeuristic impulses, transvestism, confused sexual identity, and hatred of mother, transferred to women in general, are common findings. The possibility of eventual serious attacks on women should be considered in those individuals who, in addition to burglaries, particularly burglaries committed under bizarre circumstances and alone, have a history of minor attacks on women and mistreatment of animals. The cat appears to symbolize a woman, so mistreatment of cats in combination with sexually motivated burglaries should be considered an important prognostic sign.

REFERENCES

1. U.S. Department of Justice. (1977). *Uniform Crime Reports for the Unites States.* Washington, D.C.: Government Printing Office.
2. Revitch, E. (1975). Psychiatric evaluation and classification of antisocial activities. *Dis Nerv Syst, 36*:419-21.
3. Revitch E. (1977). Classification of offenders for prognostic and dispositional evaluation. *Bull Am Acad Psychiatry and Law, 5*:41-50.
4. Guttmacher M.S. (1963). Dangerous offenders. *Crime and Delinquency 9*:381-390.
5. Banay, R.S. (1969). Unconscious sexual motivation in crime. *Med Aspects Hum Sexuality, 3*:91-102.
6. Brancale, R. Ellis A, & Doorbar, R. (1952). Psychiatric and psychological investigations of convicted sex offenders. *Am J Psychiatry, 109*:17-21.

7. Brancale, R. Vuocolo, A. McNeil, D. (1965). A profile of New Jersey sex offenders. *Welfare Reporter, 16*:3-9.
8. Revitch, E. (1965). Sex murder and the potential sex murderer. *Dis Nerv Syst, 26*:640-648.
9. Kennedy F., Hoffman H. R., & Haines, W. H. (1947). A study of William Heirens. *Am J Psychiatry, 104*:113-121.
10. Freeman, L. (1956). *Before I kill more.* New York: Pocket Books.
11. Guttmacher, M. S. (1961). *Sex offenses: The problem, causes and prevention.* New York: W. W. Norton.
12. Krafft-Ebing, R. (1965). *Psychopathia Sexualis A medico-forensics*, pp. 110-111. (H. Wedeck, Trans.) New York: G. P. Putnams Sons.
13. Revitch E. (1957). Sex murder and sex aggression. *J Med Soc NJ, 54*: 519-523.

Chapter 6

BURGLARIES WITH SEXUAL DYNAMICS

About a third of persons arrested for burglary between 1972 and 1976 were juveniles. The ever-increasing rate of burglaries throughout the years has been attested to by the successive *Uniform Crime Reports*. Thus, from 1970 to 1975 the rate of burglaries increased 40 percent in cities with populations of 250,000 and over. Seventeen percent of these offenses have been cleared by the police. The comparison of this data with the latest report from New York City (*New York Times*, July 16, 1981) indicates increases of burglaries by 6.8 percent between the first four months in 1980 and 1981, incidents rising from 81,316 to 86,866 with only 6.7 cleared by police! This data points to the growing seriousness of the problem. In spite of this, there has been a dearth of publications on burglars in the psychiatric literature.

During my association with the New Jersey State Diagnostic Center (1952-1975) I gained the impression, which I cannot substantiate statistically, that gained-motivated and drug-related burglaries have been on the increase throughout the years. In many burglaries committed by juveniles and by some adults, material gain either played a secondary role, or it was connected with emotions unrelated to what would seem to be the primary goal. Anger, depression, group involvement, the sense of mastery, importance, peers' respect derived from a successful entry, and vandalism, particularly of school property, appear to be some of the additional or main stimuli to these offenses. The motivation for burglary may be conceptualized on a spectrum ranging from professional or semiprofessional gain oriented to symbolic, subcon-

---

Source: Revitch, E. (1983). Burglaries with sexual dynamics. In L. B. Schlesinger & E. Revitch (Eds.), *Sexual dynamics of anti-social behavior* (pp. 173-191). Springfield, IL: Charles C Thomas.

sciously determined breaking and entering. In the latter, valuables or valueless objects may be removed as an afterthought or to justify and give a logical meaning to the offense. The symbolic crimes, in general, have a compelling character and most of them can be classified under the category of compulsive offenses.[1] The compulsive offenses themselves may be masked by common crime or they may be bizarre and overtly ego dystonic, or maladaptive as in Halleck's classification.[2] They may be situationally released or they may be so compelling that the offender suffers attacks of anxiety if he attempts to repress the urge. The more the offense appears to be compelling, the more one finds underlying sexual symbolism or an overt connection with sexuality.

The sexual symbolism of some cases of breaking and entry had been described previously. Banay[3] mentioned burglars who "achieve orgasm at the moment of entering a window or breaking a locked door" (p. 94). Guttmatcher[4] claimed that the personality of a burglar resembled that of a rapist and that some burglary, assaults, and cutting cases have a sexual origin. In a previous publication,[5] I described voyeuristic impulses, transvestism, confused sexuality, stealing and destruction of female undergarments, panty fetishism, in some cases masturbation while in the entered premises, connected to assault on or rape of the female occupants. In some cases, breaking and entering may precede sexually motivated gynocide. Out of 43 cases of unprovoked attacks on women including nine murders, 12 had a history of breaking and entering, with four of the 12 attacking the female occupants of the premises.[6] The well-known case of William Heirens[7,8] is illustrative. At age seventeen, Heirens entered a house through a window, removed a six-year-old girl from her bed, and cut her body into several pieces. Prior to this, he killed two women in their homes. The three murders were preceded by ritualistically committed burglaries since the age of nine years. He entered homes through the windows, experiencing excitement with ejaculation and defecation. On many occasions, Heirens tried to resist his compulsion, but this resulted in headaches, sweating, and tearing sheets off his bed. Sargent,[9] in a response to a letter to the editor concerning burglars who soil the premises, described these events as an expression of repressed rage directed at the occupants who, according to him, symbolized the offender's parents.

The following cases will illustrate the gamut of burglaries, ranging from burglaries that are gain and drug related, to the covertly and overtly sexually motivated ones. I will start with two cases, the first one mainly motivated by gain, and the second, drug related. These two cases do not exhaust all the aspects of such burglaries, but they hopefully will put the more intricate psychological aspects of sexually motivated burglars in a sharper contrast.

GAIN AND DRUG-MOTIVATED BURGLARIES

Case 1

A 25-year-old male was referred for psychiatric evaluation because he was suspected of arson, which caused the death of the occupants of the premises. While participating in burglary, the purpose of which was to steal expensive antiques, his companion and leader of the enterprise was a police officer in town. While the officer's wife detracted the home owner, an old lady living alone, by talking to her, the two men went through the dwelling and stole a few items. They opened the cellar window so that they could have an easy access to the house at night and complete the undertaking. Following the night visit, the house was set on fire, which resulted in the occupant's death.

I had the opportunity to examine I. B. 11 years previously, because of headaches, diarrhea, and poor attendance and accomplishment in school. At that time, his parents were in the process of a divorce, and I. B. was preoccupied with parental discord. Under sodium amytal injected intravenously, he revealed depressive feelings and pessimistic expectations. He was described as a quiet, withdrawn child with ritualistic, compulsive traits during preschool. In second grade, he was referred to the school psychologist for sadistic mistreatment of a smaller and weaker child. He was considered to be detached and inattentive. He dropped out of school in the eighth grade, and after holding a few inconsequential jobs, he became a car salesman. He had no record of arrests prior to the present offense, but he was previously suspected of setting a fire. This could not be proven, however.

In the interview following the burglary, he impressed me with his verbal facility and good vocabulary. He presented a façade of civility, good manners, and intelligence. A deeper inquiry, however, revealed difficulties in intimate relationships, and an episode of losing his mother and choking a woman who made uncomplimentary remarks about his sexual ineptness. The night visit of the two confederates to the old lady's house ended with her death by fire, which consumed the dwelling. I. B. was under suspicion of being responsible for the fire, but this again could not be proven.

COMMENT. The burglary of the old lady's house was primarily a gain-motivated undertaking. I. B., however, had mixed motives. He had known the confederate, whom he greatly admired, for several years prior to the incident. Without the leader's urging to help him in the undertaking, he would not have committed the crime. The fire setting could have been inspired by the leader of the undertaking as a means of avoiding detection. It is also possible that the idea originated with I. B., since he had been under suspicion of fire setting previously. Gain obviously played a main role in the enterprise, but in I. B.'s case the motivations were more complex, and thoughts of gain were intermingled with a desire to please the admired leader and with motivations of a more obscure and symbolic nature. Additional interviews, possibly with the use of sodium amytal or hypnosis, would have been necessary for deeper understanding of the hidden material.

Case 2

S. B. was 18 years old when I examined him for breaking and entering (5 counts), larceny (5 counts), and incorrigibility. He had a record of car theft, malicious damage, trespassing, disorderly conduct and illegal use of drugs. On one occasion, he had been committed to a state hospital for experiencing flashbacks connected with the use of hallucinogen drugs. Since age 15, he used marijuana, LSD, barbiturates, and, possibly, amphetamines. He admitted to burglaries of apartments and doctors' offices, specifically to steal drugs and occasionally money or valuables for the purpose of obtaining funds for his drug cravings.

All of the burglaries followed the same pattern. While his accomplices were stealing valuables, he went straight to the medicine cabinet. He described one of his burglaries as follows: "A kid told the other guys that the lady next door was rich and had gone to Florida. Four of us, including the kid, entered the house through the window. I was high on grass and I broke a window because I did not want to waste time. We took a grandfather's clock, a television set, silver, and Doriden. Doriden is all I wanted. The other kids took the rest." In another burglary he and his companions noticed a house without lights at 11:10 p.m. "One guy knocked at the door, but nobody answered. We took a window out with a butcher knife, and five of us entered the house. I went right to the bathroom. There were no drugs except for diabetes pills. My friends stole the guns and we left. We got $36 and we bought Tuinals (secobarbital sodium and amobarbital sodium).

S. B. was the only child of his parents at the time of the examination. They divorced when S. B. was 10 years old. His inability to adjust to the school routine and poor scholarship finally resulted in dropping out when he reached his sixteenth birthday. His mother applied to various agencies and to a guidance center for help, but according to her, "no one could reach the boy." On the psychometric tests, he performed within the average range of intelligence, but common sense and concept formation were reported as poor. On the Rorschach test, there was a great concern with oral gratification. His responses such as "quiet volcano," "a cat about to jump on something," and so forth, indicated a potential for explosiveness according to the psychologist. In the psychiatric interviews, he was polite and cooperative and had a warm affect. He was introduced to the drug culture at an age when he let his hair grow long so that he could gain confidence and achieve acceptance by his peer group.

COMMENT. This case illustrates a disturbed late adolescent with unstable behavior and drug dependency. The breaking and entries were clearly motivated by a desire to get either drugs, or money and valuables for their purchase.

COMPULSIVE BURGLARIES WITH COVERT SEXUAL MOTIVATIONS

Case 3

R. T., a 35-year-old prison inmate, was examined at the request of his attorney for sanity determination. R. T. committed a series of burglaries between ages 15 and 20. While on parole, after four years of imprisonment, he again, on his own admission, committed 50 to 60 burglaries within a period of six months. In early adolescence, he had been in minor difficulties in the company of his peer group, for which he was severely punished by his father. His scholastic achievement was poor and he left school at age 16. He enlisted during World War II and he was wounded in the Pacific Theater; this led to a medical discharge with a pension. His marriage after the separation from the armed services was marked by arguments, which led to an early separation. His employment history was rather hazy consisting chiefly of unskilled jobs. In addition, he started a "club with some gambling in the back."

In the interview, R. T. was friendly, with a warm affect, and was ready to discuss and reveal the most intimate fantasies and details of his life and his offenses. The description of the burglaries was vivid and detailed. The spontaneous revelations centered around four subjects: (1) the relationship with his mother, (2) his alleged generosity, (3) fantasy of finding a treasure, and (4) seeking friendship and attention. He compared his mother to Marilyn Monroe, and he talked about the apparent indifference of his half-brothers when he kissed and hugged his mother. There were indications of contributions to charitable causes, such as sending a modest sum of money for the care of a Korean child. He said that if he had been a millionaire, he would have helped "poor people, blind people, crippled people, all of them." He also fantasized "buying" an orphanage and supporting the orphaned children.

The burglaries were greatly motivated by a fantasy of finding a treasure in "cellars or in walls." He had a feeling that somewhere there was a treasure, which he had not yet found. Under hypnosis, he recollected an incident during his military service when he and his companions were swimming around a sunken ship. He then experienced a great urge to see the inside of the ship fantasying a hidden treasure. During the burglaries, he experienced a feeling of strange excitement "like walking on a tight rope" and "I can do something on my own." The tension preceding the breaking and entry was usually replaced by relaxation and triumphal feelings of "tempting the fate and being above it" when he found valuables. He admitted to voyeuristic acts in his youth, but I also learned that he had been transferred from a minimum security institution because of voyeuristic acts while there. The projective tests revealed a deep feeling of loneliness, inadequacy, and search for love and affection.

COMMENT. The spontaneous self-incriminating revelation by offenders are not infrequent.[10] Lack of direction, instability, and asocial tendencies, besides the acts of burglary, are intermingled with sentimentality and identification with the helpless and oppressed. The repeated acts of burglary have a compelling character that is connected with excitement, a triumphal feeling of mastery over fate whenever he discovered valuables, and a fantasy of eventually finding a hidden treasure. This type of triumphal feeling is more than mere satisfaction of gain. The treasure, so prominent in his ideation, is obviously a symbolic treasure. However, what does it symbolize? Does it have something in common with his voyeurism, his comparing his mother to Marilyn Monroe, a sex symbol at that time, and hugging and kissing her? In other words, are the compelling character of his acts, the excitement in entering the premises, and the search of a hidden treasure manifestations of his voyeuristic impulses? This man was examined in prison with constant noise and shouting interfering. Additional interviews with or without sodium amytal or hypnosis would have probably clarified the sexual motivation of his burglaries to a greater extent. The sexual motivation in that case would have been overt rather than covert.

Case 4

M. S., a 42-year-old convict, spent half of his life in various jails and prisons in several states, serving sentences for breaking and entering and larceny. These offenses began in adolescence. Within one month on parole, following an eight-year sentence, he was again arrested for additional episodes of burglary. According to his record, he never stayed free for more than one month between imprisonments.

A well-meaning female newspaper reporter became interested in his case, and through her intervention, he was referred to the New Jersey State Diagnostic Center, where I had the opportunity to see him on three different occasions, twice under superficial stages of hypnosis. He was not sent back–for what was supposed to be therapy–because he escaped through a window with my winter coat and gloves, unobserved by the guards, when he did not find me in the office upon his return from the men's room. He was quickly apprehended. He then presented a sorry sight, crying bitterly and looking pitifully weak and hurt.

M. S. gave a history of extreme emotional and material deprivation since his early life. Both parents were alcoholics, and his mother eventually lost custody of her younger daughter. After parental separation, the family had no sufficient food. His memories of his preadolescent years consisted of lack of food and "many times mother hollered at me for taking food out of my sister's mouth. She said the food I was eating was out of my sister's mouth. It seems there was not enough food for her and my sister. Every time I came out of the reformatory, I was blamed for eating." His work history was extremely erratic, and whenever he held a job it was only for a short time. He described himself as extremely shy, so that when his mother sent him out to look for a job, "I would say O.K., Ma, but I never went to the place. . . . When I came back, I would say I was there, and they did not take me."

The reason for much of his behavior was his inability to start a conversation or to confront people. Talking to people was accompanied by somatic manifestations of anxiety. He said that while talking to people, his hands sweat, his feet feel cold, and his heart "starts beating fast." He also complained of headaches, sleeplessness, and pain around his heart. In later years, whenever he made a date with women, he encountered in the bars, he broke into homes instead of meeting them. With the goods, he could afford to buy expensive items, which gave him a feeling of importance. "The way I looked, the money I spent there, all this made me feel important." He described himself as a very sentimental person. "I sobbed when I saw a movie about an orphanage with little children and a movie actress gave them toys. The look of the child made me cry. Another time I picked a magazine up from a table and I saw a picture of people coming from Russia to Germany. I saw everyone crying, embracing their sons and fathers. I cried and got mad at the Russians."

In a light hypnotic trance, M. S. revealed that in adolescence he used to set fires to kill cats. "I disliked cats. I would be walking the street, see cats, pet them, pick them up, and then pick up a rock, hit them on the head, and throw them into the fire. When I set fires and killed cats, I had the same feeling as when I burglarized and got jewels or hundreds of dollars. Maybe my mother liked my baby sister more, I was always alone. I always felt lonely and abandoned." Then, free associating, he suddenly said, "Once I followed a woman and hit her with a stick and then ran away. I did not want to rape her. I was not angry and I did not want to rob her, but I just wanted to hit her on the head not knowing why." He compared women with cats saying, "A cat is dainty like a woman. It keeps itself clean, washes itself. It is small. A cat has a woman's face. In fact, you can associate a woman with the cat family by their features." He expressed a great deal of resentment against his mother and added that he had started killing cats when he strongly felt maternal rejection.

COMMENT. Where as in the previous case (Case 3), the sexual motivations were implied, in this case they are more on the surface. It takes little imagination to follow the sequence of the triumphal feeling while breaking into homes instead of having a date, with the feeling of triumph in killing and burning cats, resentment of mother, and a sudden and unprovoked attack on a woman. It is of importance that he started killing cats after the experience of maternal rejection. As previously stated in this chapter, breaking and entries and unprovoked attacks on women may precede compulsive gynocide in some cases. Thus, the compelling character of his burglaries, in spite of some gain element as a motivational factor, is basically actuated by deeply-seated conflicts, with sexual connotations revolving about his mother. Additional contacts with M. S. and, very likely, psychoanalytic techniques, would add to the findings discovered in the three interviews and would clarify the connections of the various parts of the puzzle in greater detail.

COMPULSIVE BURGLARIES WITH OVERT SEXUAL MOTIVATION

Case 5

A 37-year-old male (J. J.) was referred for psychiatric evaluation following his arrest for breaking and entering, larceny, assault and battery, and attempted rape. These charges were based on the following events: Within approximately one month following his discharge from the state prison, he entered a dwelling on November 12 and grabbed a 72-year-old woman by her throat, and then, smothering her with a pillow, he either raped her or made an attempt to do so. J. J. left when the victim gave him all the money in her possession, amounting to $86. On December 2 at 6:30 a.m., he forced himself into an apartment and started choking a 67-year-old woman. He then dragged her into her bedroom, and smothering her with a pillow, he attempted to rape her. He ordered her to stick her tongue out, which she did, and then he bit it inflicting a severe wound. He allegedly told the victim that Mohammed had ordered him to kill all the white women. On December 25 at 6 p.m., he entered the bedroom of a 92-year-old woman, took $2 out of her purse and grabbed her by the throat uttering profanities. At 4 p.m. on December 26, he entered a convent, walked through the hallway to a bedroom where he placed his hand over the mouth of a sleeping nun, pulled her night dress up, and then attempted to choke her. She struggled fiercely, and he ran away when she succeeded to call for help.

J. J. had a number of arrests for robbery with firearms, breaking and entry, assault and battery, and loitering since age 15. He spent most of his life in jails and prisons. His paroles seldom lasted over a month. The offender was born out of wedlock and the whereabouts of his biological parents were unknown. He had no relatives he knew of, and the probation officer described him as "standing alone in the world." He left school in the fifth grade at age 15, but he remained illiterate. His employment history was hazy and inconsequential.

In the interviews he was shabbily dressed and unshaven. He was cooperative and polite, but detached. He spoke freely and spontaneously. J. J. could not explain the reason for his offenses, but he believed that they were gain oriented. As for his sexual history, he painted a conventional background of having sexual relations with women, masturbating occasionally and denying unusual practices. He described himself as an introvert, preferring solitude, moodiness, and being subject to diffuse headaches.

When reexamined under the influence of 500 milligrams of sodium amytal (sodium amobarbital) and 10 milligrams of methedrine injected intravenously, he said, "I want to give you all the truth, your honor. I try not to hold back nothing, if I can. I have been stealing and breaking-in all my life." He felt that he eventually would be killed and therefore he would like to spend the rest of his life in an institution. The subject matter of his spontaneous revelations dealt with sadistic fantasies and experiences, voyeuristic impulses, his attitudes toward women, and sexual preoccupations. J. J. reminisced about the killing and mistreating of animals since his childhood. Thus, he inserted fuses into horses' rectums and lit them. He cuts cows' teats off, and he wantonly killed chickens, dogs, and cats. He particularly hated cats, and in killing them he experienced a "funny feeling." A cat was the reason for one of his arrests as a juvenile. When a cat suddenly entered the room, while he was cleaning somebody's house, "I grabbed a bottle and beat and beat the cat. The man of the house tried to defend the cat." This lead to the assault on the owner of the house and the animal. He then added, "I used to kill cats with sticks, and also put firecrackers into their rectum, lit it, and let them run."

In sexual relations with women, he experienced either retarded ejaculation or could not ejaculate at all. "After intercourse," he said, "I get vicious. I then do not want to see the woman again, and I hate the world." His first attempt at intercourse was at age 24, and he defecated while ejaculating. He then had an impression that the woman either tried to kill him, or "to mess up my privates." He expressed dislike and distrust of women. He said he preferred masturbation to intercourse, since the result was the same. The only woman he ever respected was his grandmother.

He spontaneously admitted to strong urges to enter dwellings with fantasies of rape. He could not explain the impulse to bite one victim's tongue, but then, while deeply under the influence of the drugs (sodium amytal and methedrine) he said, "I wanted to see the lady's blood. I also had a feeling I wanted intercourse, but for the past five to six months, I wanted to see them bleed, but not dead." He also recollected an incident in the past when he bit a woman's nipple until it bled. At the end of the interview, still under the influence of the drugs, he asked me whether he could return for further contacts.

Nine years later, I was called to court by the prosecution as a state witness (the examination was performed at the New Jersey State Diagnostic Center) because of an attorney's request to review the case. J. J. looked much older than age 46. He was stooped, shabbily dressed, and pitiful in appearance. He not only recognized me, but he even remembered my name. He said that he did not want to leave the prison and that the idea of a review of his case was raised not by him, but by the attorney. It is of interest that on the Thematic Apperception Test (TAT) card 13 MF, he saw a man who killed his wife and was then sentenced to prison "where he is getting a rest." The Rorschach ink blots suggested to him crabs, rats, bats, and so forth. The projective tests elicited passivity, aggressiveness, poor impulse control, confusion of sexual identity, and hostility against females, thus confirming the clinical findings.

COMMENT. The sexual motives in J. J.'s repetitive burglaries were openly expressed not only in words, but also in acts. The fusion of sexuality and aggression was expressed in his desire to see women bleeding. This he accomplished by biting the tongue of one of his victims and a woman's nipple in a previous encounter. Retarded ejaculation and inability to ejaculate during intercourse may be due, among other causes, to vengefulness against a rejecting mother transferred to the sexual partner.[11] This hypothesis is quite plausible in the case of J. J. The cow and the cat are female symbols, and cutting off cows' teats and the sadistic mistreatment of cats are very suggestive of displacement of murderous aggression against women to animals. In Case 4, this transfer to a cat is quite explicit.

Case 6

A 12-year-old boy was referred for evaluation because of repetitive breaking and entries into private dwellings. This was accomplished either in the company of two juveniles or alone. W. U. took money, beer, or food if in sight, but on other occasions, he just walked through the house without taking anything, looked around, and experienced a sense of thrill and excitement. He had also stolen various items and money from his parents, and on one occasion, he attempted to remove a bag in which bus drivers deposit their fare.

On admission to the Diagnostic Center, he was originally thought to have Froehlich's syndrome, because of enlarged breasts and fat deposits in the abdomen and hips. His pubic and axillary hair, however, were fully developed in spite of his young age, and his penis looked small only because of his obesity hiding it. In early life he had had ectopic testicles, but this was successfully treated with pituitary hormones. He was described as a generally seclusive, detached, uncommunicative, and an unfriendly boy. Already at age five, he had been referred to a child guidance clinic because of restlessness and short attention span. In school he was unpopular with the peer group. W. U. hit and mistreated smaller children, and mothers in the neighborhood were constantly complaining about his behavior. In the center as an inpatient, he evidenced continuous sexual preoccupations. He was interested in pornographic pictures, he made homosexual approaches to other boys, and he propositioned two girl patients through an open window. On one occasion, he drew a penis over a boy's room. Attendants frequently found him either smoking or masturbating when alone in his room. His mother found drawings of naked women and a description of how to break a burglar alarm in his belongings.

In the initial psychiatric interviews, he was evasive and uncommunicative to a point that only some mumbling with unrevealing content was elicited. One month following his admission to the center, W. U. spontaneously revealed a dream of breaking into a store and opening the case register. In the same interview, he also described an incident when he suddenly experienced an urge to break into a house. He rang the doorbell and when no one answered, he tried to open the front door, but since it was locked, he succeeded in entering through the poorly secured back door. In the house, he opened the drawers, inspected the contents, and looked around. He left the house with a triumphant feeling of accomplishment.

Three weeks later I examined him under the influence of 7 cc of a 5 percent solution of sodium amytal and 5 milligrams of methedrine injected intravenously. Under the influence of the drugs, he was more talkative, and he spontaneously revealed the following: On one occasion, when stimulated by a picture of a woman practicing fellatio, he practiced fellatio on his brother. He frequently compared the size of his penis with his brother's. He described sexual arousal in surprising his mother taking a bath. He then had a strong urge to inspect her genitals. This revelation was followed by a period of silence. Then, all of a sudden, he said that breaking into homes is accompanied by a fantasy of finding there a naked woman. On one occasion, upon entering a house, he found a woman sleeping on the couch. He had a strong urge to lift her skirt, but courage failed him. Another interview in which he was under the influence of 6 cc of 5 percent solution of sodium amytal, was less productive. He demanded cigarettes and threatened suicide if not allowed to return home.

W. U. was the older of two siblings raised in a middle-class family. His father was described as weak. Mother was socially active and belonged to several organizations. Nine years later, when W. U. was 21 years old, he was serving a six-year prison sentence for breaking and entering and larceny, and prior to that, he served a federal sentence, but I could not determine the cause. Twenty-five years later, I accidentally found out that he was a patient in a state hospital and that he was tall and gaunt-looking rather than obese as in his preadolescence. I unfortunately could not find the reason for his hospitalization.

COMMENT. This case illustrates the necessity for painstaking investigation and prolonged observation in order to discover the hidden reasons for certain types of anti-social activities. A surface observation and examination would be sufficient to guess a serious emotional disturbance, but the sexual nature of the hidden compulsion for breaking and entries would remain undetected. Voyeuristic impulses seemed to be the main driving force. This was expressed in his fantasy to see a naked woman in the house, a sense of unexplained excitement, triumphant feeling upon entering, looking around, and inspecting the premises, and finally his urge to inspect his mother's genitals when he found her taking a bath, as well as the urge to see the genitals of the sleeping female occupant of an entered dwelling.

Case 7

A 17-year-old youth, close to his eighteenth birthday, was admitted to the Diagnostic Center on the inpatient service for evaluation of breaking and entries into homes, where he stole female underclothing and small sums of money on occasions. The first incident known to the authorities took place when he was 14 years old. At age 13, he started stealing his mother's and sister's lingerie, which he used for masturbation. He also stole female underclothing from clotheslines. At age fifteen, F. D. broke into a neighbor's house and stole female underclothing while the owners attended church services. This he planned for several days, but he could not explain the necessity for this act, since he had already an adequate supply of panties hidden in the attic for masturbatory purposes. He hid the new stolen items in the woods across the road.

Several months later, a newlywed couple moved into the neighborhood. He had seen the young lady on several occasions when he worked as a newspaper boy. At times, she came down just clad in pajamas. In the interview, F. D. described her as pretty. On the day of the offense, when he knew she was alone at home, he entered the house with a stick found in her garage. The young woman came down when she heard her dog barking. He then hit her with the stick and ran out of the house. He claimed that if he had not found her at home, he would have stolen her panties. To the arresting officer he had told, however, that his purpose was to steal her car. The episode, which resulted in his admission to the Diagnostic Center, took place under the following circumstances: The day of the incident, when both of his parents were at work, he stayed home playing his guitar and watching television instead of going to school. Stimulated by a TV show, he broke into the house of one of his female schoolmates in the neighborhood, stole her underclothing, and masturbated on the premises. While masturbating with female underclothing, he imagined having sexual relations with a girl. On occasions he imagined himself to be a girl since he thought that girls are luckier. He also mentioned dislike for girls who "tease their hair and swear and smoke."

Throughout the interviews, his affect was flat and he spoke with a sense of indifference about the various incidents. F. D. recognized the pathological nature of his drive and the necessity for change. This, however, sounded more like lip service than sincere conviction. The attendants described his behavior on the ward as "cooperative, respectful, and getting along with the peer group." On the psychometric tests, he scored within the average range of intelligence. Some of his responses to the Thematic Apperception Test (TAT) were extremely revealing. Thus, one of the cards suggested a picture of his mother dying of cancer, and another suggested his mother's ghost choking his father.

F. D. was raised in an intact working class family with a weak, passive father and an active, probably more competent, mother. None of his siblings were known to be in difficulties with the law. He had some developmental speech problems in childhood. At the time of the evaluation, he was in the eleventh grade, but his scholastic achievement was far below his grade level. He was described by his mother as being withdrawn and passive, having few friends, and having a history of truancy in school.

COMMENT. The main and overt purpose of burglaries, in this case, was to steal female underclothing for masturbatory purposes. However, the breaking into the house by itself may have a sexual connotation. In this case, he broke into the house of a newlywed with a fantasy of rape and assault, and he stated that stealing the victim's panties could have replaced the aggressive act. In another instance, F. D. actually discarded the stolen underclothing, and he planned the break-in for several days, in spite of the fact that he had a supply of panties hidden in the attic. He also disclosed transvestite and possibly transsexual fantasies, and at the same time, he expressed hostility to women and to his mother indirectly through the medium of the TAT responses and verbally, albeit obliquely, in the interview. The aggressive act and aggressive fantasies about the newlywed victim were very likely stimulated by her sexy appearance in pajamas. He placed her into the category of "girls who tease their hair and swear and smoke."

DISCUSSION

The cases presented in some detail in this chapter do not exhaust all the aspects of sexually motivated burglars. What is common in all of them is the dominance of sexual motives even if valuables and money are stolen. Voyeuristic impulses, fetishism of female underclothing, and aggression and gynocidal fantasies and acts, either alone or in combination, seem to be the most common motivating factors. On occasion, this is connected with transvestism. In a previous publication,[12] I reported the case of a 16-year-old transvestite who stole female underclothing in the broken-in dwellings and masturbated on the premises. The breaking-in by itself frequently has a sexual connotation symbolizing rape or, possibly, incest with mother. Some adolescents revealed masturbatory fantasies of breaking into dwellings. A 16-year-old youth revealed masturbatory fantasies of breaking into a store through a window. In addition, he imagined seeing his mother naked and spying on a couple engaged in intercourse through a telescope. He became sexually aroused while breaking into a store through the window, and he developed a strong urge to masturbate on the premises, but he left fearing detection.

Another 16-year-old adolescent with a history of voyeuristic acts entered a house on a sudden impulse to look around. Upon leaving, he took 35 cents out of a pile of money. This burglary obviously has nothing to do with gain, but illustrates his attempt to give a rational reason to the act. This is not uncommon in pathological offenses. The observing, the inspecting of the contents of drawers and closets, the strong feeling of curiosity and of inexplicable excitement and triumph in entering the premises, and the fantasy of hidden treasure (in Case 3) are, at least in my opinion, symbolically expressed, voyeuristic components of the sexually stimulated burglaries. In other cases, the burglar is chiefly concerned with theft of female underclothing, which he may use for masturbatory purposes as illustrated in Case 7. There are also cases of burglars ripping and destroying female garments found on the premises.

Fenichel[13] claimed that peeping may be a substitute for sadistic acting out through displacement of destructive drives by looking. Some burglaries with attacks on, and even murder of, the female occupants of the entered dwellings seem to support this assumption because of the voyeuristic component dominating in such burglaries. These attacks may also occur independently of the entries. Both types, however, are always connected with direct or indirect expressions of hatred of women. A case previously reported[6] is illustrative. Following an argument with his sister, a 16-year-old youth followed a girl on the street and hit her on the head with a stick. In the interview, he said that he was "mad at the whole female race" and that he did not care which one he hit. At age seventeen, he followed a woman on the street to her home, looked through her window, and masturbated. At age 24, he entered an apartment through the window and hit the sleeping young woman with a lead pipe. This incident occurred within four months on parole while serving a sentence for voyeuristic acts. A clear-cut connection of voyeurism, breaking and entry, and attacks on and hatred of women is obvious in this case. Case 4 in this chapter also attacked a woman with a stick without being able to explain the reason for such behavior. His hatred for women was expressed indirectly in mistreating, killing, and burning cats. He symbolically identified cats with women. This activity started when he strongly felt that his mother rejected him.

During the burglaries, he experienced the same feeling of triumph that he had in killing and burning cats. This suggests that breaking and entries, at least in this case, also have a symbolic significance of hurting or raping a woman or perhaps his mother. During World War II, I examined a 19-year-old soldier in a station hospital who had a compulsion to break into homes at night in order to hit sleeping female occupants with a stone or a brick.[12] This relieved his feelings of tension and depression. Case 5 attacked elderly women in their dwellings after a lifetime of burglaries and sadistic treatment of animals. Finally, in addition to the case of Heirens mentioned earlier in this chapter, Dr. Schlesinger reported his case of a 16-year-old youth who had a history of compulsive burglaries and sadistically murdered two women in their homes.

These cases illustrate the possible combination of burglaries and gynocidal attacks, and they suggest misogynous emotions connected with sexually motivated burglaries of all the types. Voyeuristic impulses are quite prominent in these cases. If Fenichel's assumption is correct, and destructive needs are displaced to looking, then most or all the sexually motivated burglars harbor an aggressive component in the act of breaking and entry. This component is essentially directed to mother, either in connection with incestuous strivings or as a reaction to rejection.

From mother these emotions are transferred to women in general. In a previous publication,[6] I expressed my view that the combination of breaking and entering committed alone and in bizarre circumstances, stealing of female underwear, destruction of female clothes, unprovoked attacks on women, torture and killing of cats, and expressions of hatred or contempt of women may have an ominous significance with gynocidal possibilities. Many or perhaps most of the sexually motivated breaking and entries are repetitive.

Freud's concept of repetition-compulsion, serving the purpose of repeating and thus mastering the original trauma is, at least for the time being, the only clear-cut explanation of the dynamics of the compulsive offenses. I feel, however, that in some cases, the breaking into premises with a sexual motive may be an impulsive act, very likely not repetitive and stimulated by a frustrating situation or incident. A 17-year-old youth, the son of a well-situated professional, entered a dwelling through the fire escape and disrobed in an attempt to rape the sleeping middle-aged woman. He fled the premises when she screamed. The youth was sexually inhibited and unable to experience sexual attraction to girls when close to them, but he experienced it in fantasy. The event took place following an argument with his domineering mother. Under the influence of intravenously injected sodium amytal he spontaneously recollected an incident of seeing his mother naked. This suggests deep sexual problems, very likely of a voyeuristic and incestuous nature. The psychic homeostasis was disturbed by the argument and the ensuing eruption of repressed emotions, which led to the act.

A prospective and cooperative study of such cases by several centers or individuals is a crying need. Furthermore, we have no statistical inquiries into the various types of burglaries. We are not certain about the repetition of adolescent burglaries during adult ages. The FBI, police, and particularly legal reports have no significance in the understanding of the dynamics and prognosis of such activities. My experience with such cases leads me to believe that pure legal procedures do not protect the public with deterrence or help the pathological perpetrators with rehabilitation.

REFERENCES

1. Revitch, E. (1977). Classifications of offenders for prognostic and dispostional evaluation. *Bulletin of the American Academy of Psychiatry and the Law, 5*:41-54.
2. Halleck, S. L. (1971). *Psychiatry and the dilemmas of crime.* Berkeley, CA: Univer sity of California Press.
3. Banay, R. S. (1969). Unconscious sexual motivation in crime. *Medical Aspectsof Human Sexuality, 3*:91-102.
4. Guttmacher, M. S. (1963). Dangerous offenders: *Crime and Delinquency, 9*:381-390.
5. Revitch, E. (1980). Gynocide and unprovoked attacks on women. *and Social Psychiatry, 26*:6-11.
6. Revitch, E. (1965). Sex murder and the potential sex murderer. *Diseases of the Nervous System, 26*:640-648.
7. Freeman, L. (1956). *Before I kill more.* New York: Pocket Books.
8. Kennedy, F., Hoffman, H. R., & Haines, W. H. (1947). A study of William Heirens. *American Journal of Psychiatry, 104*:113-121.
9. Sargent, D. A.: Burglars who soil premises. *Medical Aspects of Human Sexuality,* January, 1979.
10. Murphy, B. (1958). Examining the offender: Some procedures and peculiarities. *Journal of Nervous and Mental Diseases, 126*:554-567.
11. Roth, N. (1979). Sexual revenge. *Medical Aspects of Human Sexuality, 6*:8-21.
12. Revitch, E.: Sexually motivated burglaries. *Bulletin of the American Academy of Psychiatry and the Law, 6*:277-283.
13. Fenichel, O. (1945). *The Psychoanalytic theory of neurosis.* New York: W. W. Norton and Company.

Section II

MENTAL DISORDERS AND CRIME

INTRODUCTION

As an army psychiatrist during World War II, Doctor Revitch was assigned to the military disciplinary barracks in Missoula, Montana. The types of offenders whom he encountered in the disciplinary barracks left a major impression on him; in fact, he kept his notes on many of these individuals throughout his entire professional career. And he referred to his experience at the military barracks even toward the end of his life. Following the war he, like many veterans, was recruited by the Veterans Administration, and he took a job at the Lyons V.A. Hospital in New Jersey. Doctor Revitch's first published paper, "The Concept of Psychopathic Personality," which appeared in *Diseases of the Nervous System* in 1950, was written while he was on the staff of Lyons. Even though he was at a general psychiatric hospital at that time, Doctor Revitch had already developed an intense interest in the relationship between mental disorders and criminal behavior. His article on psychopathy reviewed the major published works on the topic, beginning with Prichard's (1835) *A Treatise on Insanity and Other Disorders Affecting the Mind.* He also covered the seminal ideas of Kraepelin (1913), Kahn (1931), Noyes (1944), Partridge (1928), Henderson (1947), Fenichel (1945), and Cleckley (1941).

After describing the thinking of others in the area of psychopathy, Doctor Revitch provided his own point of view, detailing diagnostic criteria that he considered to be important. Specifically, he emphasized "emotional immaturity" as the basic characteristic of a psychopath; it is manifested by egocentricity, impulsiveness, inability to form long-range plans, inability to persevere in one's endeavors, and inability to form deep feelings such as lasting friendship, love, or, for that matter, lasting deep hatred. These traits, delineated by Doctor Revitch in 1950, have been described in many contemporary works on psychopathy (e.g., Hare, 1993).

In 1952, Doctor Revitch joined the staff of the newly established New Jersey Diagnostic Center at Menlo Park. After gaining experience with sex offenders, he co-authored a paper with Doctor Rosalie Weiss on pedophilia in 1962. In it, the authors reviewed the literature on pedophilia and discussed the psychology of this type of abnormal sexual acting out. Doctor Revitch also provided his own view on the topic. He discussed his experience with older individuals who engaged in pedophilia, and he commented on states of regression, feelings of inadequacy, and interpersonal isolation as common dynamic factors. He found that the majority of pedophiles were nonviolent (other than the sex offense), and the victims were often known to be somewhat aggressive and perhaps even seductive in their own way.

After 25 years of experience with various forms of criminal behavior, Doctor Revitch developed a method of classification of offenders for prognostic and dispositional assessment. In a paper on this method, he described a motivational spectrum with external, or sociogenic, stimuli on one end and purely internal, or psychogenic, stimuli on the other end of the hypothetical continuum. He emphasized how an individual's level of personality integration, empathic capacity, and value system are important factors in the overall assessment of offenders. He also discussed and described catathymic and compulsive offenses and emphasized that these offenders need to be studied and carefully monitored because the source of the problem is internal.

In 1979, Doctor Revitch wrote a fascinating paper on patients who kill their physician. The impetus for the paper was a case he had involving an individual who killed his psychiatrist; the homicide was perhaps triggered, in part, by the physician's cold and somewhat rejecting and abrupt interpersonal behavior. The paper reviews the scant literature on the topic, which emphasized that this type of murder is relatively rare. Doctor Revitch noted that the paranoid and the depressive with chronic medical complaints are the types of patients who might act out in a violent way, with the paranoiac heading the list by far. Urologists and proctologists–because of their dealings with areas of sexual significance–are the most likely medical specialists to be killed by a patient. Curiously, Doctor Revitch noted that a malpractice suit against the physician may absorb the paranoid patient's rage and thus decrease the likelihood for assault on the doctor. He emphasized that physicians need to be readily available to patients as a means of preventing not only suicides but many malpractice suits and violent or homicidal assaults as well.

The last three papers in Section II deal with Doctor Revitch's original concept of conjugal paranoia. The notion of conjugal paranoia--a specific type of paranoia with encapsulated delusions and pathological attitudes directed against the marital partner--has been considered a major contribution to the field. In fact, the *Diagnostic and Statistical Manual of Mental Disorders-III's* definition is right out of Doctor Revitch's paper (unfortunately without attribution): "[In] delusional jealousy ('conjugal paranoia') . . . an individual may become convinced without due cause that his or her mate is unfaithful. Small bits of 'evidence,' such as disarrayed clothing or spots on the sheets, may be collected and used to justify the delusion" (American Psychiatric Association, 1980, p. 195).

Doctor Revitch noted astutely that often the paranoid partner in a marital situation may appear healthier than his or her mate, and the illness will not be detected by a superficial or cursory evaluation. A significant amount of time has to be spent with the paranoiac, as his or her ideation will often leak out; this ideation is initially characterized by humiliating and destructive acts against and ideas regarding the spouse. These ideas and behaviors may precede the outbreak of a full paranoid delusion. Individuals with conjugal paranoia often have good contact with their surroundings, and they are able to conduct their affairs very well. Doctor Revitch emphasized that the best diagnostic tool is "an unhurried and careful interview of both spouses by the same psychiatrist." He concluded that individuals who develop conjugal paranoia are inadequate and emotionally weak people with confusion in sexual identification.

Doctor Revitch co-authored an article with John W. Hayden, who, at the time, was a student at Rutgers Law School. The paper appeared in the *Rutgers Law Review* in 1955. Doctor Revitch and Mr. Hayden presented the concept of conjugal paranoia, guidelines on how to recognize a paranoid litigant, and problems the attorney might encounter in handling paranoiacs as both plaintiffs and defendants. This fascinating article is as relevant today as it was in 1955 and should be read carefully not only by mental health professionals but by lawyers, judges, and, particularly, matrimonial attorneys who may come in contact with these difficult individuals.

The last chapter in Section II deals specifically with the differential diagnosis and disposition of paranoid marital partners. In this brief paper, Doctor Revitch discussed the difficulty in diagnosis, common symptoms, and how paranoiac individuals in marital relationships can be extremely difficult to manage. He made a sharp distinction between individuals who are pathologically jealous and those with a clear encapsulated paranoid delusion, a psychosis. Pathological jealousy occurs in insecure individuals, and psychotherapy may be successful with them. Conjugal paranoia, however, has a poor prognosis, and separation of the marital partners should be recommended in most cases. Doctor Revitch again cautioned against misdiagnosing the healthy spouse as the one who is paranoid or mentally ill.

REFERENCES

American Psychiatric Association. (1980). *Diagnostic and statistical manual of mental disorders, III.* Washington, D.C.: American Psychiatric Press.

Chapter 7

THE CONCEPT OF PSYCHOPATHIC PERSONALITY

Prichard[1] in England in 1835 was the first to attract the attention of the medical world to a condition he termed "moral insanity" or "moral imbecility" and which he described as follows:

> "There is a form of mental derangement in which the intellectual functions appear to have sustained little or no injury, while the disorder is manifested principally or alone in the state of the feelings, temper and habits. In cases of this nature, the moral or active principles of the mind are strangely perverted or depraved; the power of self-government is lost or greatly impaired and the individual is found to be incapable, not of talking or reasoning upon any subject proposed to him, but of conducting himself with decency and propriety in the business of life."

In the latter part of the nineteenth century, Krafft-Ebing[2] in Germany, and Bianchi[3] and Tanzi[4] in Italy described cases seldom treated in hospitals, but who are characterized by complete insensibility and absence of moral judgment and ethical notions. Koch[5] in 1888 introduced the concept of constitutional psychopathic inferiority, including hysteria and obsessions in this entity. Kraepelin[6] described constitutional psychopathic states and psychopathic personality. In the former, he included sex deviates, psychasthenics, as well as nervous and despondent individuals. In the latter group, he included cases described by Prichard, "born" criminals, morbid liars and swindlers. Kraepelin

---

Source: Revitch, E. (1950). The concept of psychopathic personality. *Diseases of the Nervous System, 11*:1-4.

hinted at a possible relationship of psychopathy to psychoneurosis and psychosis.

In spite of the many papers and books written on the psychopathic personality, the definition and the psychopathological concepts vary with the authors and, therefore, the diagnosis of psychopathic personality is still considered a wastebasket of psychiatry. Some of the authors are mentioned here because their concepts have become classical.

Eugene Kahn[7] in 1931 defined psychopathic personality as a descriptive term indicating inadequate social functioning which is a result of quantitative changes of impulse, temperament and character. According to Kahn, personality is determined by the three above-mentioned functions. Under impulse, he understands conative forces which are genetically determined; temperament which is composed of affect and mood, which also are genetically determined; character which is comprised of striving toward a goal, attitude toward oneself and people, and it is socially determined.

Noyes[8] defined the psychopathic personality as "various inadequacies and deviations in the personality structure of individuals who are neither psychotic nor feebleminded, the defect existing primarily in the conative, emotional and characterological aspect of the personality. In spite of deviations, there is no loss of synthesis of the personality like in psychosis."

Partridge[9] defined psychopathy as a lack of socialization and he prefers the term "sociopathy" to psychopathic personality. He emphasizes that there are various degrees of sociopathy and quantitative differences which shade over into the normal.

Cleckley[10] in his book *Mask of Sanity* described the psychopathic personality as an individual devoid of human emotions, as a "robot of indescribable ingenuity, who is able to do everything that a whole and healthy personality can do except participate in life on a personality level." He compares the psychopathic personality to a "psychobiologic machine, a machine that appears to be a whole personality but actually is moved by something very different." The actions and emotions of a psychopathic personality are mechanical and devoid of depth.

Henderson[11] has an all embracing concept of psychopathy. According to him, the psychopathic state is characterized by instability, queerness, explosiveness, intuitiveness and egocentricity. He included in this category men of genius and people like Joan of Arc and Colonel Lawrence.

The psycho-analytic school itself has not formed a concept acceptable to all the psychoanalysts. Thus, Ben Karpman[12] feels that most of the patients diagnosed as psychopathic personality are in reality neurotics or schizophrenics. A true psychopathic personality is, according to Karpman, a constitutional state, characterized by an inability to form ethical standards or a super-ego. He claims that after years of analysis, no psychogenic source for the condition can be found. He prefers the term "anethopathy" to psychopathy and he uses the term anethopath in describing what he calls a true psychopathic personality. Lindner[13] in his book *Rebel Without a Cause*, asserts that psychopathy is a disorder of behavior which affects the relationship of the individual to his social setting. The conflict with society results from psychosexual immaturity, for the psychopath never develops beyond the pregenital stage, and therefore, perseverance, planning and gradualness are impossible. In his own case, having gone through hypno-analysis, Lindner claims to have found a memory of the primal scene he had witnessed at the age of six months, which he considers a traumatic event.

Fenichel[14] stressed that psychopathic personalities are unable to direct their actions toward a positive aim of achieving a goal. Their actions are directed toward the negative aim of getting rid of tension. A psychopath is like an infant who had not learned to coordinate purposeful movements nor to postpone immediate desires. Like in an infant, tension is felt as a threat to existence and has to be relieved without postponement. For this reason, he calls psychopathy an impulse neurosis.

Some psychiatrists question the very existence of psychopathy and they believe that psychopathic reactions are usually manifestation of either schizophrenia or psychoneurosis. All functional psychiatric disorders can be reduced to a form of reaction to anxiety. Therefore, if one followed the logic of these psychiatrists, they would classify all non-organic reaction types as anxiety states. Our diagnostic criteria are based more on symptomatology than on dynamics and, therefore, certain types of immature, asocial individuals should be placed in a separate category. It is admitted that this category is ill-defined, that it merges on the one side with schizophrenia and psychoneurosis and with simple immaturity and egocentricity on the other side; that psychopathy is essentially a sociopathy and that there are various degrees of psychopathy and quantitative differences between so-called normal individuals and typical psychopaths. However, every sociopath cannot indiscriminately be classified as a psychopathic personality, for sociopathy is frequently an expression of psychoneurosis, early schizophrenia or criminality.

Although various personality disturbances may frequently be responsible for criminal behavior, it is very often determined by the social environment and moral values and concepts conflicting with the established patterns. On the other hand, one should be careful of not missing a psychopath merely because of record of good conduct and adequate army service. We believe that emotional immaturity is the basic characteristic of a psychopath. This immaturity is manifested by egocentricity, impulsiveness, inability to form long range plans and to strive toward definite goals, inability to persevere in one's endeavors, inability to form deep feelings such as lasting friendships, love, or for that matter, lasting deep hatred. We agree with Fenichel that the psychopath, like an infant, is unable to handle tension in a realistic way and that he is forced to release it without delay. Hence his inability to conform to the reality principle; his impulsiveness, and frequently his moodiness and his escape mechanisms such as malingering, alcoholism, drug addiction, and at times hysterical manifestations and psychotic breakdowns, are all symptoms.

The ethical standards or super-ego of the psychopath was the first to attract the attention of the early observers. Certainly, the super-ego of the psychopath is weak. This, however, is not a primary inborn or constitutional characteristic as suggested by Karpman, rather it is a result of emotional immaturity. In our opinion, psychopaths without any trace of a super-ego are extremely rare. What we feel is true, is that their ethical feelings are superficial, as superficial as their total affectivity. They may rejoice or grieve with somebody, but this will not be lasting. They may feel indignant over unethical acts, but this indignation will lack depth of feeling. This superficiality of emotional life gives us an impression of a "psychobiologic machine that appears to be a whole personality, but actually is moved by something very different," as expressed by Cleckley. It is not surprising that the behavior of this type of individual is frequently, but not necessarily, sociopathic. Another common manifestation of a psychopath's immaturity is his tendency toward histrionics, to show off, to be in the limelight. Often psychopaths will make unsuccessful suicide attempts in certain situations in order to attract attention, just another way to be in the limelight or to escape unpleasant, tension producing situations.

Is it possible for a psychopath to have neurotic and psychosomatic manifestations? Certainly, it is possible and many of them show manifestations of anxiety. There is no reason why the same individual should not have neurotic and psychopathic traits combined, although some psychiatrists feel that psychopaths "act out" their conflicts, whereas neurotics "act in" their conflicts.

Sexual deviates, alcoholics, and drug addicts are frequently classified as psychopaths. Many psychopaths may revert to alcohol and drugs to relieve their tension. Thus, we feel that only sex deviates should be classified as psychopaths who, in addition to their deviations, show immaturity traits described above.

As for etiology, the theories can be divided into constitutional, organic, and psychological. Constitutional defect was stressed by older investigators. That is why psychopathic personality was called constitutional psychopathic inferiority or constitutional psychopathic state. The modern theories tend toward the psychological view, stressing disturbed family environment in early childhood. It is known that some cases of head injury, Sydenhams's chorea, and epidemic encephalitis are followed by sociopathic behavior, and many observers, including Nielsen[15] feel that in many cases an organic basis can be found in psychopathic personalities. This view seems to be substantiated by several electroencephalographic studies where abnormal records were found in a large proportion of cases. However, Knott and Gottlieb[16] found that abnormal EEG's are more frequent in psychopaths with a neurologically loaded family history and past personal history of head trauma or severe illness.

SUMMARY

The historical background of the concept of psychopathic personality and the present day views were given. Although the very existence of this entity is denied by many psychiatrists, it is felt that individuals whose basic symptomatology is manifested in the sphere of social relationships and whose basic psychopathology is manifested by immaturity reactions, should be classified as psychopathic personality. Most modern investigators support psychological theories of the etiology of psychopathy. The older investigators believe that it is a constitutional disease and some modern investigators feel that in many cases it may have an organic background which seems to be substantiated, to some extent, by abnormal electroencephalographic records.

REFERENCES

1. Prichard, J. L. (1835). *A treatise on insanity and other disorders affecting the mind.* London: Sherwood, Gilbert & Pifer.
2. Krafft-Ebing, R. von (1886). *Psychopathia sexualis*, Philadelphia: F. A. Davis.
3. Bianchi, L. (1906). *A textbook of psychiatry.* London: Bailliere, Tindall & Cox.
4. Tanzi, E. (1909). *A textbook of mental diseases.* New York: Rebman.
5. Koch, J. L. (1888). *Psychopathic inferiorities*, Ravensburg, Germany: Dorn.
6. Kraepelin, E. (1913). *Lectures on clinical psychiatry* (3rd ed.). New York: William Wood.
7. Kahn, E. (1931). *Psychopathie.* Berlin, Germany: Gruyter.
8. Noyes, A. P. (1944). *Modern clinical psychiatry.* Philadelphia: W. B. Saunders.
9. Partridge, G. D. (1928). A study of cases of psychopathic personality. *American Journal of Psychiatry*, 7:953-974.
10. Cleckley, H. (1941). *The mask of sanity.* St. Louis, MO: C. V. Mosby.
11. Henderson, D. K. (1947). *Psychopathic states.* New York: Norton.
12. Karpman, B. (1948). The myth of the psychopathic personality. *America Journal of Psychiatry*, *104*:523.
13. Lindner, R. M. (1944). *Rebel without a cause.* New York: Grune & Stratton.
14. Fenichel, O. (1945). *Psychoanalytic theory of neurosis.* New York: Norton.
15. Nielsen, J. M., & Thomson, G. N. (1947). *Engrammes of psychiatry.* Springfield, IL: Charles C Thomas.
16. Knott, J. R., & Gottlieb, J. S. (1944). EEG evaluation of psychopathic personality. *Archives of Neurology and Psychiatry*, *52*:515.

SUPPLEMENTAL REFERENCES

1. Bromberg, W. (1949). Emotional immaturity and anti-social Behavior. *J. of Clinical Psychopathology*, *8*:424.
2. Cason, H. (1948). Characteristics of the psychopath. *Am. J. of Psychiat.*, *105*:211.
3. Gilbert, G. M., Goering, H. (1948). The amiable psychopath. *J. of Ab. & Sco. Psychol.*, *43*:211.
4. Gottlieb, J. S., Ashby, M. D., & Knott, J. R. (1946). Primary behavior disorders and psychopathic personality. *Am. J. of Neurol. & Psychiat.*, *56*:381.
5. Greenacre, P. (1945). Conscience in the psychopath. *Am. J. of Orthopsychiatry*, *15*:495.
6. Preu, P. W. (1944). The concept of psychopathic personality. *Personality and Behavior Disorders, Vol. II*, page 922. New York: The Ronald Press.

7. Ripley, R. S., & Wolf, S. (1948). Psychoses occurring among psychopathic personalities in association with inelastic situations overseas. *Am. J. of Psychiat., 105*:52.
8. Silverman, D. (1943). Clinical and EEG studies of criminal psychopaths. *Arch. Neurol. & Psychiat., 50*:18.
9. Silverman, D. (1944). The electroencephalogram of criminals, Analysis of 411 cases. *Arch. Neurol. & Psychiat., 52*:38.
10. Simon, B., O'Leary, L., & Ryan, J. J. (1946). Cerebral dysrhythmia and psychopathic personality. *Arch. of Neurol. & Psychiat., 56*:677.
11. Simmons, D. J., & Diethelm, O. (1943). EEG studies of psychopathic personality. *Arch. of Neurol. & Psychiat., 55*:619.
12. Solomon, H. C. (1948). Adult character and behavior disorders. *J. of Clinical Psychopathology, 9*:1.
13. Solomon, J. C., & Yakovlev, P. L. (1943). *Manual of Military Neuropsychiatry.* Philadelphia, PA: W. B. Saunders Co.
14. Stearns, W. (1944). Unfit personalities in the military service. *Personality and Behavior Disorders, Vol. II.* New York: The Ronald Press.
15. Weiss, I. I. (1946). Rehabilitation of military offenders at the 9th service command rehabilitation center. *Am. J. of Psychiat., 103*:172.
16. Weiss, I. I. (1947). Psychosis in military prisoners. *J. of Clinical Psychopathology, 8*:689.
17. A Compendium of neuropsychiatry in the Army. (1943). *The Army Medical Bul., No. 66*:1.

Chapter 8

THE PEDOPHILIAC OFFENDER

Pedophilia is an adult's sexual attraction to physically immature children of the same or opposite sex. Men and women may indulge in pedophiliac activities; however, our experience has been limited to adult males. The male pedophile may exhibit his genitals, kiss, caress, and touch the body of the victim, commit fellatio on boys, cunnilingus on girls, or reach a climax through noncoital relations such as rubbing genitals against the body of the child or inducing the child to manipulate his genital parts. Coital relations with penetration are uncommon, and rape, rape-murder, and lust-murder are extremely rare.

The rarity of serious sexual aggressions against children is supported by Guttmacher[1] in the following excerpt: "Fortunately child murders are rare. Because each case is given nationwide press coverage and because of the great emotional impact of these horrible outrages they seem to be much more frequent that they are." Since a recent rape murder of a four-year old child by a pedophile aroused a wave of public concern and anxiety, it may be timely to present our experience with pedophiliac offenders examined at the New Jersey State Diagnostic Center.

Under the New Jersey Sex Offender Act, all persons convicted of certain sex offenses are committed to the New Jersey State Diagnostic Center, Menlo Park, New Jersey, for a psychiatric-psychological evaluation. As of April 1961, over 4,000 sex offenders have been examined in the out-patient clinic at the Center. In a tabulation of the first 1,206 sex offenders at the Center,[2] it was found that 327 (27.1%) committed offenses against adolescent victims from 13 to 15 years old, 314 (26%)

Source: Revitch, E. & Weiss, R. G. (1962). The pedophiliac offender. *Diseases of the Nervous System, 23*:73-78.

against children from 7 to 12 years old, 71 (5.9%) against children under the age of seven years, and 124 (10.3%)) against children of an unspecified age. The total number of offenses against children under 16 years old was 836 (69.4%).

In the tabulation of 329 sex offenders examined between July 1, 1960 and April, 1961, 219 (67%) were involved with children under 16 years old. Lafon et al.[3] and Deshais[4] indicated that 75% of the sex offenses in France, and 65% in the department of Mayenne were committed against minors. Krafft-Ebing[5] referring to the French statistics in 1885 and 1892 also reported the frequency of child victims of sex offenders. Therefore, it appears that the prevalence of children as victims of sexual offenses is an old universal problem rather than a new local phenomenon.

The frequency of older age groups in sexual offenses against children was mentioned by various authors. Karpman[6] quotes the findings of the Mayor's Committee that older men tend to molest young children, while Guttmacher[1] quotes the findings of the Los Angeles Police Department which reveals that the mean age of a rapist is 23 years, while the mean age of sex offenders against children is 41 years.

The authors conducted a study at the Diagnostic Center which compared the age relationship between the sex offender and his victim. The victims were classified from three to 11 years representing the prepuberty group, and the victims from the 12-to-15-year age range were classified as the preadolescent and adolescent group. The adult offender groups were classified as young adults (16-24), adults who passed the average age for marriage (25-52), and the older adults (53-76) who passed their climacteric. As shown in Table 8.1, the older men have a predilection for physically immature children, while the adolescents and emotionally immature young adults are usually involved with children from 12 to 15 years old.

Table 8.1
PSYCHOLOGICAL AGE OF SEX OFFENDERS AND THEIR VICTIMS

	Age of Offenders			
	16-24	25-52	53-76	Total
Age of Victim	11.40%	37.00%	64.00%	N = 62
3-11	88.60%	63.00%	36.00%	N = 157
12-15	N = 88	N = 117	N = 14	N = 219

Chi-square = 25.31 (.01 level of significance).

The young offender should not be classified as a pedophile since the age difference between him and his victim is negligible. In homosexual offenses committed by preadolescents and young adolescents on children, the indulgence in fellatio is indicative of homosexual fixation, while forcing the victim to commit fellatio or to submit to rectal intercourse may be just a part of adolescent maladjustment and aggressiveness.

We rarely had the opportunity of examining the victims of pedophiles; however, we have the clinical impression that quite often the child victim is aggressive and seductive and sometimes induces the adult offender to commit the offense. Our impression is supported by Karpman[6] who quotes various authors indicating that children with attractive personalities and concomitant behavior difficulties are frequently involved with pedophiles, and he feels that quite often the child victim is a victim in the legal sense only. Rogers and Weiss[7] found that in a study of 59 girls and 15 boy victims under 15 years old, the degree of their participation ranged from simple compliance with the offenders' wishes to actual solicitation of his sexual advances. These victims were classified as participating victims by the authors, while those victims who appeared not to have participated were called accidental victims.

The participating victims were of the lower socioeconomic level, emotionally deprived, and had a stronger need for approval. In quoting the Michigan report of 1951, Karpman indicates that 72 percent of the victims were known to the offender. Weiss et al.[8] found that of 73 girl victims, only 11 were involved with strangers, while 62 were involved with neighbors, friends of the family, and members of the family. The frequency of involvement with neighbors and friends of the family corresponds to our own clinical impression.

Classification

It is difficult to find a common denominator as a basis for classification of pedophilia, but the three following categories seem to emerge:

1. Choice of object according to sex
2. Nature of pedophiliac act
3. Personality and mental state of the offender

1. **Choice of Object According to Sex**. The pedophiliac acts may be classified as heterosexual and homosexual. The heterosexual acts are far more common (80.7%) than the homosexual offenses (19.3%) according to the tabulation of the first 1206 cases at the Diagnostic Center.[2]

2. **Nature of the Pedophiliac Act**.
(a) Noncoital: Contacts with the child include oral copulation, kissing, caressing, and fondling the genitals of the victim, or having the victim perform these acts on the offender, and emission through rubbing genitals against the body of the child.
(b) Exhibitionism: Most exhibitionists linger in the vicinity of schools, playgrounds or parks, and expose themselves to immature children usually of the opposite sex.
(c) Coital Contacts Without Violence: Sexually mature girls between the ages of 13 and 15 are more likely to indulge in sexual relations with late adolescents and young adults than with older pedophiles. Coital contacts are rare with children under the age of 12 years.
(d) Coital Contacts with Violence: This category includes rape, rape-murder, and lust-murder. These offenses are comparatively infrequent, although they have been recorded in the literature. The best example of lust-murder on a large scale is the historical case of the French nobleman Gilles de Ray, who in the fithteenth century tortured and murdered in his castle an estimated 800 children. DeRiver[9] cites the case of a 32-year-old married male who visualized immature girls while having sexual relations with his wife. He planned his crimes by winning the children's confidence and then raped and killed them. Children may also be accidental victims of violent acts by polymorphously perverse pre-psychotic and psychotic individuals. One of the best examples is that of Heirens,[10] who in 1945 murdered and dismembered a six-year-old female child. However, Heirens also compulsively murdered two older women, burglarized numerous homes, and was a panty fetishist.

3. **Personality and Mental State of the Offender**. The pedophiliac offenses may consist of a fixed, compulsive, repetitive pattern, or of impulsive acts of a situational nature. Although there is

> no clear-cut boundary dividing the groups, a division into compulsive and impulsive-situational behavior has a practical value for prognostic reasons. Our experience shows that pedophilia is most likely to occur in certain types of personality organizations. It is more common in those individuals who are emotionally immature, physically underdeveloped, or have physical and mental defects. Pedophilia is also likely to occur in individuals who are in states of regression such as loss of potency, alcoholic inebriation, and early senility.

The early senile pedophiles warrant a special mention. Krafft-Ebing[5] mentioned a reawakening of sexual impulses in older people before the appearance of a well-defined manifestation of intellectual decline. In our experience, 8 out of 219 pedophiliac offenders examined between July 1, 1960 through April 1961, fell in the age range of 60 to 76 years, and they showed no classical symptoms of senile psychosis such as deterioration of recent memory. In many instances, the senile pedophiles are still bright and alert, but there may be a general deterioration of habits connected with loneliness and various frustrations of old age.

Psychology of Pedophilia

The predominance of the older age group, and the people with various physical and mental defects among the pedophiles, suggests that pedophilia is essentially a regressive state and retreat from adult challenges. The theory that the heterosexual pedophile feels uncomfortable with adult women, and is therefore attracted to immature girls, is supported by many authors dealing with the subject. Krafft-Ebing[5] stated that a common factor concerning pedophiles and their acts is that they are "childish, unmanly, knavish, and often silly."

According to Hirschfield,[11] pedophiles and gerontophiles are psychosexually infantile and pedophiliac acts are in reality sexual games of children. Bromberg[12] states that the mainspring of pedophilia is to be a child again and the anxiety regarding potency and inferiority feelings leave them to seek younger children in order to save their ego. Karpman[6] quotes Hirning as saying that sex offenses against children all have in common some fundamental organic or functional psychopathology which prevents the individual from seeking sexual contact with mature individuals of either sex.

As a rule, pedophiles like children, frequently consort with them, and in spite of the great disparity in their age differences, enter into a peer type of relationship with them. The precocious and aggressive children quickly sense the infantile characteristics of the adult pedophile, and very soon they lose the awe of adult authority, and the children treat him as if he were one of them. The pedophile will complain that the children annoyed him, that they followed him into the bathroom when he had to urinate, and that they exploited him through accepting his gifts and money, which he allegedly distributed just because of friendly feelings or in order to help a deprived child. It is true that gifts may occasionally be distributed to entice a child into sexual activity; however, we feel that the non-coital sexual contacts are more frequently a consequence of the peer relationship than of gifts and bribes.

On many occasions, the pedophile feels lonely and deprived so that contact with the child gives him a feeling of closeness and warmth. Hammer[13] et al. claim that "intense loneliness causes the pedophile to seek children as easier individuals than adults to whom to relate." Fenichel[14] states "usually love for children is based on a narcissistic object choice. Unconsciously the patients are narcissistically in love with themselves as children." In our experience, the majority of heterosexual pedophiles seek out children for sexual gratification because of personality inadequacies. However, in homosexual cases, the seeking out of a child has more of a compulsive component, and Fenichel's assumption of narcissistic love seems to be more common. The homosexual pedophiles are often attracted to positions which bring them in contact with young boys, and through constant contact with the youngster an emotional attachment, as well as noncoital contacts, may take place. We could not find any cases of female pedophilia in our records but this does not mean that such cases are nonexistent or rare.

CASE HISTORIES

Five cases are presented. They do not exhaust all the aspects of pedophilia. We attempt to illustrate states of regression and feelings of inadequacy and isolation present in many pedophiles. In the homosexual Case, 5, we attempt, in addition, to illustrate the mechanism of fixation and narcissistic identification.

Case 1 – Senile Pedophilia

A 67-year-old ex-Cossack officer who escaped from Russia during the Revolution came to the United States a few years after World War II. While living with his step-daughter in a Russian refugee section, he was apprehended for having non-coital relationships with two girls, 7 and 8 years old. The act involved touching the lower part of the body of the children and having them place their hands on his penis.

In the interview, he was well oriented in all spheres. He became tearful when the examiner (Doctor Revitch) conducted the interview in the Russian language. He then displayed a military decoration he had received during World War I and said he was a hero and no one here recognized his past deeds. He said with tears in his eyes that he was going blind and only his prayers to St. Alexander Nevsky saved his eyesight. He then fell on his knees making the sign of the cross and asking for help. He tearfully denied his offense and blamed the children's father for plotting against him.

He was seen several months later in a prison hospital where he was treated for a large hernia. He recognized his former examiner (Doctor Revitch) and his memory seemed to be intact; however, his judgment was more impaired than before. He was worried about his military decoration which had been taken to the prison office and, in a mixture of Russian and broken English, he attempted to explain to other amused inmates how he had led an attack on a Turkish position during World War I.

Although this patient does not show the typical memory defect of senile psychosis, he exhibited personality changes characterized by regressive features in the emotional sphere and by poor judgment. However, some of his actions could be ascribed to cultural conditioning. Senile changes enhanced by life difficulties and social degradation were basically responsible for this regression and its sexual expression.

Case 2 – Pedophilia with Organic Defect

A 26-year-old male was arrested for touching little girls in their neighborhood. Since this type of behavior continued after he received some psychotherapy, he was finally committed to a state hospital. His developmental history and clinical findings are typical of the brain damaged group of patients. Born by breech delivery, as a baby he had difficulty in swallowing milk. He did not sit up until one-year-old, his speech remained defective, and his motions were clumsy and poorly coordinated. Some degree of athetosis and facial grimacing were noted and he also had a club foot. He was not retarded, as he had a Full Scale IQ of 106 as measured on the Wechsler Adult Intelligence Scale. In spite of his handicaps, he had two years of college and held a job for a short time. He lived with his overprotective parents.

He would spend several hours in the bathroom every morning indulging in excessive masturbation while conjuring images of "improperly" dressed young girls. He claimed that the children he touched were "improperly" dressed. He never had sexual relations or dates with adult women. It is obvious that in this case his physical handicaps and unfavorable appearance created a poor self-image and prevented normal contacts with the opposite sex. A child was less of a threat to his ego.

Case 3 – Pedophilia with Exhibitionism

A 39-year-old male was referred to the Diagnostic Center after conviction for public lewdness. He had exposed himself before small children in the playground. He has spent some time in a state hospital previously for similar offenses. He was short, toothless, untidy, and disheveled. The offender spoke hurriedly in an indistinct whining voice. There were no psychotic manifestations. His history revealed emotional and material deprivation since childhood. His father was an alcoholic and his stepmother beat him and openly favored her own children. In his youth, peers made fun of him because of his shabby clothes. He felt lonely and inadequate. He made a good adjustment in military service during World War II, but after discharge, he felt "dizzy, weak, and nervous." He held many unskilled jobs, such as a dishwasher.

The offender married a mentally defective woman but the marriage lasted only a few months. In the interview, he expressed a need for love and acceptance. Tearfully he said, "I want a wife . . . a home . . . good food. I don't want to get into trouble. I wouldn't hurt kids. I wouldn't rape a girl. I like kids. People don't know how I suffer. There is nowhere for me to turn, yet I am as smart as people who went to high school. I want a wife to work for me, to take care of me, but I have no luck." He said that he masturbated instead of approaching women for sexual satisfaction. He liked to watch children at play and this somehow stimulated him to exhibit his genitals.

The projective tests revealed a weak, submissive, hypochondriacal person with homosexual conflicts. This patient is more disturbed than the average pedophile since he presents distinct schizoid traits. He has the usual feelings of inadequacy as a male and strong dependency needs. The only adult woman he approached and married was mentally defective. He felt content when he was with the children on the playground, but even here he needed vicarious satisfaction through exhibiting his genitals and masturbating. No doubt the visit to playgrounds was also a search for closeness and an attempt to get out of isolation.

Case 4 – Pedophilia with Coital Relations

A 47-year-old widower was apprehended in his trailer having sexual relations with an 11-year-old girl. The girl had been abandoned five years before by her parents and the patient had been given her custody. When the child came to live with him, he stopped all outside activities and interests. At the time, she was undernourished and had no decent clothes. He provided her with all the necessities and recollected in the interview how "her eyes were brilliant when she asked whether the clothes were really hers." The patient satisfied his sexual urges through masturbation, visualizing adult women he saw on the street. However, the closeness of the child induced a feeling he remembered as follows: "As I can remember, I played with the child. I loved her and I still love her. It is hard to put into words what was going on in my mind. Maybe we lived too close to each other. When I was at work, I was just wondering where she was. She was my love and I would give my life for her."

The child frequently sat on his lap which induced him to pet and kiss her. When she was eight years old, he put his hand on her genitals and this produced an emission. A few months later they started to have sexual relations. In the patient's life history, there was a great deal of affective and material deprivation. In the interim, he was depressed expressing numerous hypochondriacal complaints. He revealed a feeling of loneliness and isolation, and he stated that for the past several years he was unable to carry on a conversation. Consequently, he gave up all of his associations, and the little girl filled the void.

Case 5 – Homosexual Pedophilia

A 23-year-old man was treated by the examiner (Doctor Revitch) for a period of one and a half years because of homosexual interests in pre-adolescent boys. He was first examined after telling a neighbor that he used to peep through a window, while standing on a ladder, just to observe a pre-adolescent boy in the nude. When he was between six and seven years old, he used to daydream about a boy classmate being naked. He had no recollection of other sexual fantasies until he entered high school. At this time, he experienced a desire to touch and fondle the genitals of other boys. In his masturbatory fantasies, he visualized naked boys. One of his pastimes was to trace naked bodies over pictures of boys in magazines. He always had been seclusive, moody, and subject to short periods of depression. His classmates constantly teased him and this contributed to his feelings of apartness and isolation.

His mother was an attractive self-centered woman who left her husband when the patient finished high school. The father, an engineer, was well-meaning, but uncommunicative. In college, the patient first tried to major in Ancient Greek, but after 1½ years of study experienced a feeling of futility. He became seclusive and was unable to concentrate which made it necessary for him to give up school and return home.

He rapidly improved with supportive psychotherapy. During this course of therapy, a girl cousin moved into his father's house because of an out-of-wedlock pregnancy. The patient and this cousin had been intimate once as children when he was 14 and she was 11. The intimacy had consisted of her placing her hands on his genitals while she was naked, causing him to have an erection which frightened him. However, during the course of therapy, he became enamored and had sexual relations with her. During this time, his homosexual fantasies were completely abandoned. After she gave birth to a child, the cousin moved to a distant state and he again became attracted to young boys.

The patient was in trouble again when he lured a 10-year-old neighbor's son into his room and grabbed the boy's genitals. He later claimed that the act was impulsive and that he entertained a thought, at that time, to strip the boy naked. He disclosed fantasies of being a girl and of being ashamed of having a large penis. In discussing his feelings which led him to commit the offense, he stated, "I was envious of him. I wanted to be him rather than myself. In him, I saw freedom. He seemed to be happy and I admired him. I mostly wanted to feel him or to masturbate him. I wanted to give him something so that he would be obligated to give me friendship in return." Later, he disclosed masturbatory fantasies involving a handsome boy in sexual play with an attractive girl. He identified himself with the handsome boy who was so attractive that girls ran after him and seduced him. He claimed that his ultimate object was heterosexuality, but being unable to attain it on his own, he attained it through identification.

This patient can be classified as an incipient ambulatory schizophrenic. His psychosexual development was thwarted to the extent that infantile sexuality dominated even in masturbatory fantasies. Fenichel's[14] assumption that love for children is a narcissistic love of oneself as a child, is amply illustrated in this case. Homosexuality in this case seems to be a flight from heterosexuality. Yet, through identification, he vicariously indulged in heterosexual play. Not all homosexual pedophiles present a picture as complex as this patient. In many instances pre-senile or senile subjects or alcoholics may indulge in homosexual relations with children when their sexual prowess is on the wane or when they feel alone or isolated.

SUMMARY AND CONCLUSIONS

Pedophilia is a sexual attraction to physically immature children. The problem is of importance, since the majority of victims of sexual offenders are below the age of 16 years. Aggressive acts and coital relations are rare. The offenses usually consist of various noncoital contacts. Prevalence of older age pedophiles was noted by many authors, and this observation was verified by the Diagnostic Center research. States of regression, feelings of inadequacy and isolation are the most common dynamic factors. In some cases, particularly in homosexual pedophiles, fixation and narcissistic identification can be elicited. The majority of pedophiles are passive individuals and their victims are usually known to be aggressive and sometimes seductive children. Our experience is limited to males, although female pedophiles are mentioned in the clinical literature of sexology. We have had little experience with therapy in this area; however, we feel that the senile pedophiles and pedophiles with schizoid and regressive features, will not respond well to psychotherapeutic endeavors. For these cases, we recommend hospitalization.

REFERENCES

1. Guttmacher, M. S. (1951). *Sex offenses: The problem, causes and prevention.* New York: W. W. Norton & Co.
2. Brancale, R., Vuocola, A., & MacNeil, D. (1954). *Diagnostic Center Report.*
3. Lafon, R., Trivas, I., & Pouget, R.: Aspects psychologiques des attentats sexuels sur les enfants et les adolescents." *Ann. Med. Psycholog., 116*: 865-897.
4. Deshais, G. (1954). Les reactions anti-sociales dans la mayenne. *Ann. Medico-Psycholog., 112*:192-211.
5. Krafft-Ebing, R. V. (1934). *Psychopathic sexualities.* New York: Physicians and Surgeons Book Co.
6. Karpman, B. (1954). *The sexual offender and his offenses.* New York: Julian Press, Inc.
7. Rogers, E., & Weiss, J. (1953). Study of sex crimes against children. (pp. 47-53) *California Sexual Deviation Research.* Department of Mental Hygiene, State of California, Jan.
8. Weiss, J., Rogers, E., Darwin, M., & Dutton, C. (1955). A study of girl sex victims. *Psychiat. Quart., 29*:1-27.
9. DeRiver, P. (1949). *The sexual criminal.* Springfield, IL: Charles C Thomas.
10. Kennedy, F., Hoffman, H. R., & Haines, W. (1948). Psychiatric study of William Heirens. *J. of Crim. Law and Criminology, 38*:311-341.
11. Hirschfield, M. (1944). *Sexual anomalies and perversions.* London: Francis Aldor.
12. Bromberg, W. (1948). *Crime and the mind.* Philadelphia, PA: J. B. Lippincott Co.
13. Hammer, E., & Glueck, B. G., Jr. (1957). Psychodynamic patterns of sex offenders. *Psychiat. Quart., 31*:325-345.
14. Fenichel, O. (1945). *Psychoanalytic theory of neurosis.* New York: W. W. Norton & Co., Inc.

Chapter 9

CLASSIFICATION OF OFFENDERS FOR PROGNOSTIC AND DISPOSITIONAL EVALUATION

The purpose of a psychiatric examination of offenders is for the determination of legal responsibility, fitness to stand trial, and for the prognosis and dynamic factors leading to the offense. Prognosis is closely tied in with the dynamics of the offense and with the offender's personality organization in terms of ego strength, fantasy life, value system and empathic capacity. The psychiatric diagnosis per se, without the evaluation of the factors mentioned, is usually unrewarding. The disposition of the offender depends, at the present, more on legal than on psychodynamic and predictive considerations, unless the offender is officially declared insane in accordance with a legal formula. According to Sadoff,[1] "Too much print and time has been spent on responsibility and competency, and precious little energy has been expended by lawyers and psychiatrists working together to help solve dispositional and predictive problems in the criminal law. Hopefully this imbalance will soon be corrected." This paper is written in the hope of making a modest contribution toward the correction of this imbalance.[1]

The consensus is that the prognosis of dangerousness is tenuous and unreliable.[2-4] Tanay[5] states, "The description of a tendency is frequently confused with prediction of the occurrence of a future event like homicide or suicide." In other words, the prediction of dangerousness and of recidivistic acts is not on a yes or no scale, but on a scale of a tendency and a probability. The problem of dangerousness and

Source: Revitch, E. (1977). Classification of offenders for prognostic and dispositional evaluation. *Bulletin of the American Academy of Psychiatry and Law,* 5:41-50.

recidivism is frequently confused with the prognosis of a mental illness. Rubin[3] states, "It is not always possible to establish a connection between mental illness and the nature of crime." The confusion about this connection was well-illustrated in the following New Jersey case:[7]

Case 1

A young black man entered the police station and shot and wounded the officer at the desk. This happened shortly after race riots in the town. The young man had a history of treatment in a mental hygiene clinic since childhood. In jail, following the incident, he developed an acute schizophrenic reaction with catatonic features, and therefore he was transferred to a state hospital. He was declared insane at the time of the offense under the McNaghten Rule, but following his improvement with electroshock therapy, a question of release contingent on dangerousness was raised. In deliberations, the Superior Court of New Jersey emphasized "neutralization" of the patient's condition and questioned the ability of the psychiatrists to predict psychotic episodes in the future. No consideration was given to the dynamic factors leading to the offense or to the fact that a prognosis of the illness is not identical with the prognosis of the offense.

The only offenses whose prognosis and direct causation are identical with the diagnosis of the illness are cases of paranoid schizophrenia in which the delusions and hallucinations influence the commission of the act. There are also very rare cases of violence committed during attacks of psychomotor epilepsy, in states of post-ictal confusion or in toxic confusional states. The best example of a crime committed under the influence of paranoid delusions is the case of Daniel M'Naghten himself, who killed the private secretary of Sir Robert Peel in 1843.[7] Another illustration is the following case:

Case 2

A 15-year-old boy described as quiet, withdrawn, and self-conscious killed two little girls six and seven years old. The victims' bodies were found in a wooded area behind their homes where they had been playing. Their heads were crushed and bodies beaten. In spite of the fact that he was considered mentally retarded in childhood, his full scale IQ on the WISC was 108. The Rorschach responses were bizarre. The

TAT responses were replete with violence and a feeling of victimization. In the interview, he stated that his peers disliked him and that he heard the voices of his tormentors calling him names such as "pussy." He developed a hatred for his peers, and to relieve his feelings he, at times, threw rocks at trees. On the day of the offense, while walking alone, he suddenly heard the two little girls laughing. At this point he said, "I jumped . . . they were laughing . . . then I heard the voices of the kids calling me names." He was markedly improved when reexamined five years later. Vagueness, incoherence, and hallucinations elicited previously were no longer detected.

It was obvious that at this point he was no longer dangerous, since his offense was a direct outcome of his mental condition. Accordingly, some sort of classification based on a common denominator underlying the various offenses is necessary. Prior attempted classifications tended to divide the offenses according to the nature of the crime, according to the psychiatric diagnosis, and according to legal considerations. For instance, Brancale[8] proposed two classifications, an administrative and a psychiatric. In search of a dominant pattern, he divided his psychiatric classification into a normal group, a deficit group, a neurotic reactions group and psychotic reactions group. Each group had many subdivisions, thus complicating the issue. This classification is chiefly based on psychiatric diagnoses. Clark's[9] classification is based on the nature of the criminal act. He divided offenses into (1) white collar crime, (2) organized crime, (3) crime in the streets, (4) crimes of passion, (5) violation of regulations, and (6) revolutionary crimes of terrorism. This classification is completely devoid of dynamic and predictive elements.

Halleck[10] comes closer to the deeper dynamics of criminal behavior, as he divided crime into (1) adaptive and (2) nonadaptive. Adaptive crime is committed for some rational, self-serving purpose, while nonadaptive crime is actuated by emotional conflicts. It is obvious that the nonadaptive crime has psychiatric implications while the adaptive crime is sociologically determined. Tappan,[11] in reviewing psychiatric classifications of delinquency, mentioned Franz Alexander's and Hugo Staub's scheme proposed in 1931. This classification is based on a combination of psychiatric and motivational factors. Thus the offenders are divided into (1) acute criminals whose offenses are accidental, (2) chronic pseudosocial criminals whose offenses result from social factors, (3) neurotic criminals whose offenses are determined by psychological factors, and (4) pathological criminals whose offenses are a consequence of an organic brain disease. Thus, it seems that some students of criminology, such as Halleck, Alexander and Staub, recognize exogenous and endogenous factors in the causation of criminal behavior and classify offenses accordingly.

During my twenty three-year association with the New Jersey State Diagnostic Center--whose function was to evaluate juvenile delinquents, sex offenders, criminal cases, cases of marital difficulties, and various other behavioral problems referred by courts, institutions and agencies–it was not the psychiatric diagnosis or the nature and the legal aspect of the offense, but the motivational stimuli leading to the act which were important.[12] The exogenous sociogenic and the endogenous psychogenically determined offenses are distributed along a motivational spectrum with the purely exogenous at one extreme and the purely endogenous at the other. In moving from the exogenous to endogenously stimulated offenses, the spectrum is divided into (1) environmental offenses, (2) situational offenses, (3) impulsive offenses, (4) catathymic offenses, and (5) compulsive offenses. I have slightly modified the scheme from the original paper[12] in placing the catathymic offenses ahead of the compulsive offenses. It is obvious that no classification of behavior can be or should be rigidly pigeonholed, since we are dealing with a continuum and not with hermetically closed categories. This condition implies borderlines with characteristics belonging to the adjoining areas.

A. Environmental Offenses. The present rise in crime is primarily due to social and environmental influences. A combination of social pressures and weakening of social controls is responsible for this phenomenon. Rapid social changes, economic deprivation, and sense of alienation provide the background for the events. There are many historical examples which demonstrate that the weakening of authority and discipline by itself may create social disintegration and produce disorganized antisocial behavior. The most recent examples include the newspaper reports of looting and crime in civil-war-torn Beyrouth and indiscriminate murder under the guise of ideology in Northern Ireland. Another historical illustration was graphically presented by Wedgewood[13] in her book on the Thirty Years' War. The undisciplined and demoralized mercenary armies ravaged the countryside and committed all kinds of indignities against the local population. The importance of social organization and attitudes of leaders in group conduct was also illustrated by Storry[14] in his history of Japan. Thus, the Japanese Army treated the local population and war prisoners gallantly during the Russu-Japanese War of 1904-1905, while in the climate of World War II, the overrun populations and prisoners of war were treated with inhumanity and indignity. The My Lai massacre had definitely something to do with the moral climate of the war, which very likely released homicidal cravings of the accused.

The climate of either the lack of authority, or of authority permitting and abetting cruelty, will release sadistic needs of predisposed individuals who otherwise would live normally in a civilized environment. A perfect example is supplied by the surviving Nazi war criminals who in a peaceful environment in exile committed no crimes. Adolph Eichmann[15] is an example. According to the reporter who interviewed the Israeli psychiatrist assigned for the pretrial evaluation of Adolph Eichmann,[16] he impressed one as a "simple, ordinary man." Yet, additional interviews and projective tests disclosed a great many underlying murderous desires. The young man reported in Case 1 spoke about black-white antagonism as his motive for shooting the police officer. This general antagonism, however, was just a vehicle and direction for the release of aggressive tensions.

The majority of environmentally stimulated offenders are nonpsychotic and with a fair personality organization. Sutherland's[17] theory of differential association (i.e. criminal behavior as learned in interaction with others) generally applies to this group. The most striking examples are participants in organized crime. The following case is illustrative:

Case 3

The patient was a low-ranking figure in the organized crime system. He was a married man supporting his family and speaking fondly of his children. In the interview, his affect was warm; he was friendly and he spoke freely and volubly. His wife was sitting in the waiting room with the federal agents who brought him in for examination. In talking about his extra-marital affairs, he wanted to make certain that his wife could not hear him. He was raised in an economically deprived working-class family. At the age of 14 years, he was induced to steal cars and to perform other services for the petty neighborhood gangsters. From petty thefts, he graduated to bigger jobs, and later on he committed murders by orders of his superiors. He viewed the criminal activities as a job, and this, he felt, was completely separate from his private life and from his religious and ethical feelings. He had typical middle-class ambitions for his children and he did not want his daughter to marry into a crime family. As he grew older, he was developing a resentment toward his crime organization, feeling that he was chained to the organization. He described his road into organized crime through youthful realization that his life could be richer and brighter if he accepted a different set of values. He said, "As a kid I was deprived. My father worked hard for a living. There was no money in the house. Other kids ate steaks, we ate macaroni."

The prognosis of this individual depends entirely on the structure of his social environment. It would obviously be favorable if his organization could be liquidated and organized crime in general checked.

B. Situational Offenses. Situational offenses are in essence reactions to stressful situations. They are mostly committed by individuals with no or little psychopathology, although all sorts of personalities can be involved. Two of the best descriptions of situational offenses can be found in Theodore Dreiser's *Sister Carrie* and in his classic *An American Tragedy.* In *Sister Carrie,* a business executive, unhappy with his family life, falls in love with a young girl, a recent arrival in town. This involvement led to divorce proceedings, resulting in economic loss and finally in a state of depression. In this state, he finds the business safe open, which he was supposed to check at the end of the day. He caught sight of "a layer of bills in the safe." This vision resulted in the following experience as described by the author: "Count them" said a voice in his ear. He put his hand into the first of the boxes and lifted the stack, letting the separate parcels fall. They were bills of fifty and one hundred dollars, done in packages of a thousand. He thought he counted them such. "Why don't I shut the safe?" his mind said to itself. "What makes me pause here?'" For an answer there came the strangest words. 'Did you ever have ten thousand dollars in ready money?" This money could solve his present predicament and allow him to live with Carrie. He had been a reliable and trustworthy employee prior to the event.

I had an opportunity, during my assignment to the U.S. Disciplinary Barracks in World War II, to examine many cases of situationally precipitated murders. A minor disagreement, fear or anger, resulted in shooting or stabbing the opponent, with whom the offender seemed to be on friendly, or at least on neutral terms prior to the incident. The following case is illustrative:

Case 4

A 22-year-old soldier of average intelligence (full scale IQ 108 on the WAIS), with a history of adequate civilian and army adjustment, participated with his friend in the killing of a homosexual. The offender was stationed at the time in a wild, isolated area in New Guinea. He and his friend were under the influence of liquor when a homosexual soldier offered to perform fellatio for a fee. The friend accepted the offer, but refused to pay. This started a fight during which the homosexual was killed. It was a situational offense connected with pent-up emotions due to their service in a wild, isolated tropical area, with an emotional release influenced by alcohol, along with the hostile attitudes of the immature toward homosexuals.

C. IMPULSIVE OFFENSES. Impulsive characters react with antisocial acts in certain situations. The offenses are of a diffuse, poorly structured, unpremeditated or partially premeditated stimulus-response nature. They differ from the situational offenses by the multiplicity of antisocial acts and in their poor impulse control. The life pattern of these offenders is characterized by looseness of personality integration, lack of direction, and unpredictability. A previously reported case[12] involved a 19-year-old youth with a history of various juvenile offenses, including vandalism, breaking and entering, and use of drugs. While babysitting for his sister, with his 19-month-old niece, he raped her rectally, stimulated by the sight of her buttocks. This resulted in the child's death. In this case, the offense was a clear-cut stimulus-response act. In most of the impulsive offenses, the stimulus-response quality is not as immediate as in this case. The following case is illustrative:

Case 5

A 25-year-old man was referred for sanity determination by his attorney. He was a suspect in the murder of his girlfriend's estranged husband. The suspect had a long history of juvenile delinquency, use of drugs, and adult offenses consisting chiefly of breaking and entering. He spent time in juvenile and adult correctional institutions and also had several admissions to psychiatric hospitals. His employment was sporadic. Once, while working as a guard, he stole explosive sticks from the company which employed him at the time. He threw the sticks into a lake, causing an explosion. The offender had a tendency to tell exaggerated, self-incriminating tales of his crimes, and he was beset by grandiose and aggressive fantasies.

He gave the following account of the last incident. He was in a pizza parlor with his "fiancée" when suddenly he felt like seeing if someone he knew was in the tavern next door. He told his fiancée he was just leaving her for a short time to buy cigarettes. In the tavern, he was introduced to the estranged wife of the victim. He took his fiancée home and returned to the tavern. He told his new girlfriend that he was a triggerman (one of his exaggerations). She asked him to get rid of her husband. He obtained a gun, but it is not clear whether he or his new girlfriend of one week pulled the trigger.

In the interview, the offender spoke clearly and he was very cooperative. His judgment was quite defective, yet there were no overt psychotic manifestations. He remarked that he was a model of behavior in institutions, but upon release something happens to him. He said he does not know why he gets into trouble. It is obvious that this person needs structure and guidance for normal functioning. Without a structured environment, be becomes a victim of chiefly exogenous, but also endogenous stimuli.

D. Catathymic Offenses. The term *catathymia*, coined by H. W. Meier,[18] who described "psychic disorders marked by perseveration in the course of which a single depressive topic tends to be complex-determined." Gayral et al.[19] described "*crises catathymique,*" as emotional outbursts of a psychogenic and organic origin, presenting a differential diagnosis with psychomotor epilepsy. I described, under the name catathymic, severe emotional outbursts in a prison population.[20] However, it was Wertham who introduced the concept of "catathymic crisis" as a diagnostic category into psychiatric criminology. Wertham[21] originally defined his concept as follows: "A catathymic reaction is the transformation of the stream of thought, as the result of certain complexes of ideas, that are charged with a strong affect, usually a wish, a fear or an ambivalent striving." Various modifications of the original definition can be found in his subsequent publications.

I believe that Wertham's "catathymic crisis" is not a diagnostic entity, but rather a psychodynamic process characterized by an accumulation of psychic tension in connection with some conflictual relationship. This process may be acute, of very short duration, leading to a sudden unexpected violent outburst, or a chronic, slowly developing process, lasting many months. In both forms, the acute and the chronic, superficially integrated individuals, but secretly struggling with feelings of inadequacy and particularly sexual inadequacy, resort to violence when the potential victim challenges the offender's sense of integration, adequacy or sexual competence. Violence, usually resulting in homicide or some destructive act, serves the purpose of freeing oneself from the source of threat to the psychic homeostasis. The act may be followed by a sense of relief.

In the chronic catathymic process, depressive mood and schizophrenic-like thinking may precede or accompany the violent act. A good description of the chronic catathymic process can be found in Yukio Mishima's *Temple of the Golden Pavilion.* The following two cases are illustrative of an acute and a chronic catathymic process.

Case 6

A 30-year-old teacher, without a history of previous offenses, killed a seven-year-old girl when she rang his doorbell to sell brownie cookies. Since she had no change for a 20-dollar bill, she offered to return later. He suddenly felt angered and humiliated by the offer. He then ordered her to follow him into the cellar and to undress. When she complied, he attempted intercourse, but due to premature ejaculation he failed to consummate the act. He then battered her, and when he realized she was dead, he calmly put the body in a plastic bag and disposed of it far away from home in a wooded area. The offender lived with his mother and grandmother. Sometime before the event, he had been engaged, but for some reason broke off the relationship. The day of the offense he was depressed and felt lonely and inadequate. It was a holiday and some of his colleagues took a short trip. He was invited to join them but he refused, although he wanted to go.

In the face-to-face interview and in the interview under the influence of intravenously injected sodium amytal, his affect was flat and he expressed no emotions. There were no overt psychotic manifestations such as delusions, hallucinations, disturbance of associative processes, or intrusion of bizarreness into his thinking. On the surface, he made an adequate social and work adjustment. However, a great deal of self-doubt and feeling of sexual inadequacy could be unearthed in the interviews.

Case 7

This following case was reported in full previously.[22] It illustrates the chronic from of the catathymic process. A 22-year-old man killed his girlfriend with multiple stab wounds during a car ride. While stabbing her, he also kissed her, and when she fell dead to the floor his first impression was that she was joking. The murder was preceded by several months of vague homicidal and suicidal fantasies. He mentioned these thoughts to a friend and to his minister, but his warnings were not taken seriously. These thoughts seemed unreal to him. Three weeks prior to the incident, he drove to the future victim's home with a loaded gun. This event was perceived as an unreal and dreamlike experience. He felt relieved after the arrest since "I do not have to worry about her anymore."

In the interview, his thinking was loose. He cited the *New Testament* and expressed guilt over having had sexual relations with her rather than guilt over the murder. He compared his act with Abraham sacrificing Isaac. He was charged with first degree premeditated murder and sentenced to life imprisonment. Before the trial, he mentioned, "They all think that I planned it. It was just in my mind. I never thought it would happen." A psychologist who saw him recently in the state prison (about 15 years after the incident) described him to me as bizarre and deteriorated.

I testified at the trial that he was an insidious schizophrenic who fell apart during, and due to, the relationship with his girlfriend. It seemed to me that he should have been treated as insane, in conformance with the M'Naghten Rule. In my experience, the jury considers most of these cases as sane and their acts as premeditated.

E. Compulsive Offenses. The compulsive offenses are on the endogenous end of the motivational spectrum. They are entirely determined by inner psychological sources with virtually no or little environmental influences, except for the cases whose antisocial compulsions, normally dormant, are released either through sanctions from authority, or by permissiveness and disintegration of the social order. Obviously compulsive offenders of the latter type have a better personality organization than the compulsive offenders whose fantasies break through without environmental stimuli. The compulsive offenses may be committed in a specific, ritualistic manner, or they may be of a more diffuse nature, but with an underlying common need variously expressed. Fantasies may precede the offenses by many years. In one of my cases, the tying of women's legs with a rope was preceded by 31 years of fantasying the event.[23] Therefore, people with sadistic and homicidal fantasies should be taken seriously. The offenses may be repeated quite frequently once they start, as in the cases of Heirens[24] and the Boston Strangler,[25] but they also may occur only once or at intervals of many years.

The literature and clinical experience are filled with examples of bizarre murders, assaults, and fire-settings for which the offenders served long sentences, and then performed similar acts while on parole. In my own experience, a young man who was condemned to death for the brutal killing of a high school girl (but whose sentence was commuted to life imprisonment), attacked a woman with a knife many years later while on parole. The urge to commit the act may be so overpowering that the offender experiences severe anxiety if he abstains. Thus, Krafft-Ebing,[26] reporting the case of a patient (Case 3) who had a compulsion to stab women in the genitals, described his attempts to abstain in the following words: "For a while he succeeded in mastering his morbid cravings, but this produced a feeling of anxiety, and copious perspiration would break out from his entire body." The following two cases are representative of a ritualistically executed compulsive offense (Case 8), and one of a more diffuse offense expressing a compulsion to hurt women (Case 9).

Case 8

A 19-year-old soldier examined on the prison ward of an army station hospital duri-ng World War II had a compulsion since the age of 12 years to break into homes at night, to enter the bedroom, and to hit the sleeping woman with a brick or a stone. When overcome by the urge, he would usually drink beer in order to gain courage. His offenses were committed in a similar ritualistic manner.

Case 9

A 37-year-old man was convicted of attempted rape, breaking and entering, larceny, and assault and battery. He had a number of arrests since his adolescence for robbery, assault and battery, and breaking and entering. Within one month after his release from the last imprisonment, he entered a dwelling and raped a 72-year-old woman. Three weeks later, he forced his way into another dwelling where he choked and raped a 67-year-old woman. A few weeks later, he entered a convent and attempted to choke a nun with a pillow while she was sleeping. When interviewed under the influence of sodium amytal injected intravenously, he begged for help and he revealed various sadistic acts such as cutting cows' teats off, putting explosives into horses' rectums, and killing animals in a sadistic manner. He expressed distrust of women and an extreme dislike for cats. He also expressed a desire to remain in a prison or in any other institution for the rest of his life.

SUMMARY AND COMMENT

In an attempt to find a common denominator for prognostic and dispositional classification of offenders, it seems that the psychiatric diagnosis and the legal implications are of less significance than the motivational stimuli leading to the offense. Thus, the motivational stimuli are grouped spectrally with sociogenic on one end and purely endogenous, psychogenic stimuli, on the other end of the scale. This category does not include offenses due to overt paranoid delusions or to organic confusional states. In addition to the motivational stimuli, one has to evaluate the personality integration, the empathic capacity, and the value system of the offender. The situational offenders have the best prognosis. The catathymic offenders have a much better prognosis than the compulsive and impulsive offenders, while the prognosis for the environmental offenses depends to a great extent on the value system of the offender and on further opportunities to commit crime. As to disposition, it is clear that the impulsive, catathymic and compulsive offenders cannot be deterred by legal measures and that specialized, psychiatrically guided, institutions are necessary for research, handling, and treatment of these cases. Situational and particularly environmental offenders should be treated in the traditional correctional manner, unless they are mentally incompetent and ill.

REFERENCES

1. Sadoff, R. L. (1975). *Forensic psychiatry.* Springfield, IL: Charles C Thomas.
2. Dershowitz, A. M. (1973). Dangerousness as a criterion for confinement. *Bull Amer Acad Psychiat Law, 2*:172-179.

3. Rubin, B. (1972). Prediction of dangerousness in mentally ill criminals. *Arch Gen Psychiat, 27*:397-409.
4. Researchers challenge prediction of dangerousness in offenders, pp. 13-19. *Psychiatric News*, Dec. 3, 1975.
5. Tanay, E. (1975). Dangerousness and psychiatry. *Current Concepts in Psychiatry, 1*:23.
6. *New Jersey v. Carter*, 64 N. J. 382 (1974).
7. Tuke, D. H.. (1967). The McNaghten rule. *Documentary History of Psychiatry*, Goshen C. E. (Ed). New York, NY: Philosophical Library.
8. Brancale, R. (1955). Problems of classification. *National Probation and Parole Association Journal, 1*:118-125.
9. Clark, R. (1971). *Crime in America*. New York, NY: Pocket Books.
10. Halleck, S. (1971). *Psychiatry and the dilemmas of crime*. Berkeley, CA: University of California.
11. Tappan, W. P. (1949). *Juvenile delinquency*. New York, NY: McGraw-Hill.
12. Revitch, E. (1975). Psychiatric evaluation and classification of antisocial activities. *Dis Nerv Syst, 36*:419-421.
13. Wedgewood, C.V. (1969). *The Thirty Year War*. New York, NY: Penguin.
14. Storry, R.(1972). *A History of Modern Japan*. New York, NY: Penguin.
15. Wilson, C., Pitman, P. (1962). *Encyclopedia of murder*: New York, NY: J. P. Putnam.
16. Explorations of the mind of Adolf Eichmann. *Medical Tribune*, Nov. 26-27. 1966.
17. Sutherland, E. H. (1947). *Principles of criminology*. Philadelphia: Lippincott.
18. *Dorland's Illustrated Medical Dictionary* (25th ed.), (1974). W. B. Saunders.
19. Gayral, L., Millet, G., Moron, P., Turnin, J. (1956). Crises et praoxysmes-catathymymiques. *Ann Med Psych, 114*:25-50.
20. Revitch, E. (1964). Paroxysmal manifestations of non-epileptic origin: Catathymic attacks. *Dis Nerv Syst, 22*:662-669.
21. Wertham, F. (1937). The catathymic crisis. *Arch Neurol Psychiat, 37*:975.
22. Revitch, E. (1965). Sex murder and the potential sex murderer. *Dis Nerv Syst, 26*:640-648.
23. Revitch, E. (1957). Sex murder and sex aggression. *J. Med Soc New Jersey, 14*:519-523.
24. Freeman, L. (1956). *Catch me before I kill more*. New York, NY: Pocket Books.
25. Ray, G. W. (1967). *Confessions of the Boston strangler*. New York, NY: Pyramid.
26. Krafft-Ebing. (1934). *Psychopathia Sexualis*, New York, NY: Physicians and Surgeons Book Company.

Chapter 10

PATIENTS WHO KILL THEIR PHYSICIANS

The purpose of this paper is to warn physicians that they may become the target of homicidal assault by a disgruntled patient. Urologists and proctologists who deal with the genital organs and the anal orifice are the most likely to arouse the suspicion and anxiety of paranoid patients. Retribution for real or imaginary injustices, allegedly perpetrated by the physician against patient, is the leading motive. The physician may have treated the assailant for a number of years or may have had little direct or indirect contact. Heads of institutions or chiefs of services may become the primary target. Two types of patients are likely to kill their physician: paranoid patients and depressives with vague, continuous hypochondriacal complaints. Paranoids head the list.

CASE PRESENTATION–A. B.

Several years ago, the author was asked to examine A. B., a 53-year-old man for sanity determination. His history indicated that he had entered, unscheduled, the office of his psychiatrist and sat patiently in the waiting room for about two hours while the physician was treating other patients. Finally, when called into the office and told that it would be a short visit, he shot the doctor in the chest, killing him on the spot. Following the murder, he surrendered to the police.

The murderer was the psychiatrist's patient for a period of 13 years for treatment of depression. During that time, A. B. had been hospital-

---

Source: Revitch, E. (1979). Patients who kill their physician. *Journal of the Medical Society of New Jersey*, *76*:429-431.

ized for electroshock therapy on three occasions. The killing took place within three to four weeks following the last hospitalization.

The patient was a machinist with high school education, who always supported his family. His own early life was marked by poverty with severe emotional and material deprivation. His father was an abusive alcoholic who eventually died in a mental hospital. The patient was of normal intelligence with a full scale IQ of 107 on the Wechsler-Bellevue Intelligence Test. Since the test was given within approximately two months following the last electroshock treatment, it is quite probable that he had a higher intellectual endowment because of reversible memory impairment usually caused by this therapy. Lack of confidence, depression, perfectionistic concerns, and looseness of thinking were elicited on the projective tests.

In the psychiatric interview, A. B. was cooperative and extremely appreciative of the attention given to him. He felt he needed help. His speech was coherent and logical. He was well oriented and he could give his life history and the course of events leading to the homicidal act with clarity and in good chronological order. There was no evidence of delusions, hallucinations, or paranoid thinking. He was known as a very accurate worker, to a point that his employer once remarked that he was "too fussy" with his work. On this occasion, possibly because of low mood and the effect of electroshock therapy, his performance was criticized. Over the weekend, he brooded over his "failure," and the day of the incident he resigned from his job over the objection of his employer. He then proceeded to the doctor's office.

A. B. later said that he did not intend to kill the doctor, but just to have him suffer "as I suffered." The killing, he felt, was a "mistake." His account of his relationship with the psychiatrist was interspersed with descriptions of incidents he interpreted as rejection and lack of interest. This, however, was always followed by some statement exonerating the doctor. He hoped for a closer relationship with his doctor. "I expected more of him. He was really not concerned and I felt there was no personal interest." The offender spoke a great deal about the deprivation in his childhood and he recollected that he had never received money from his parents for ice cream. He also disclosed resentment against his father. A. B. believed that he would finish his own life as his father did, in a mental hospital. The court considered the patient insane at the time he committed the offense and committed him to a mental hospital under the purview of the McNaughten Rule.

REVIEW OF THE LITERATURE

Very little has been written about the specific problem of patients killing their physician. Dupré[1] classified these patients as "persecutes-persecuteurs" (persecuted persecutors) in a paper he presented to the Société-Médicopsychologique July 16, 1918 on the occasion of the murder of a Professor Pozzi by a patient on whom he had operated for varicocele. The patient committed suicide following the shooting of the surgeon while the latter was sitting in his office. In a review of the then available literature on the subject, Dupré referred to the case reported by Legrand du Saulle in his 1877 treatise of legal medicine. The case is so illustrative that it deserves to be mentioned in full translation.

> A coachman named Bourgeois, who had been treated by our colleague, accused Dr. Bleynie of mishandling his `cold in the intestines.' He complained of an illness which resisted the treatment by Dr. Fiévé for sixteen years. This hypochondriac then consulted Dr. Bleynie, who ordered hot baths followed by bathing in the river. He then consulted Dr. Biett in the hospital St. Louis in Paris, and steam bath was suggested. The suffering of our insane increased and he then declared that the treatment had dessicated his intestines, and he accused the physicians of torturing him and causing an incurable condition. He then decided on revenge and he killed Dr. Blynie with two shots from his pistole. (Legrand du Saulle, 1877)

Another typical case mentioned by Duprè was Doctor Guinard, a surgeon at the Hotel Dieu in Paris, who was killed by a patient on whom he had performed an operation for a "chronic affection of the anus." Alliez and Savy[2] reported more recently the killing of a physician by a foreign worker employed in France. The physician had seen this patient only on one occasion. The patient failed to fill the doctor's prescription, believing that it contained poison, and that the victim of his assault planned to have him expelled from the country.

In the case when the homicidal patient attacks the physician in the emergency room or in his office, Frazier[3] recommends the approach of "talking down an armed patient in violent crisis." According to him, confrontation in an open hallway rather than in a closed room is preferred. The "talking down" takes a long time and "it takes more staying power than bravery." Madden and Lion[4] warned clinicians to be sensitive to the precursive signs of possible assault such as agitation, threatening verbalizations, and gestures.

DISCUSSION

The murder of a physician by his or her patient is relatively rare, but such as eventuality cannot be discounted. Most of the murders and harassment of physicians are committed by their paranoid patients. Paranoid phenomena can range over a wide spectrum of clinical conditions from major paranoid psychosis, to a paranoid syndrome secondary to the psychogenic and organic conditions.[5] Paranoid personalities are prime candidates for dissatisfaction with medical care. Procedures involving the genitalia and excretory system may lead to malpractice actions or to assaults on the physician. A paranoid patient may become violent in the middle of a sigmoidoscopic examination.[6] Not all paranoids are overtly and recognizably psychotic. The paranoid projections may be interpreted by observers as true statements when they are not bizarre in content. Furthermore, they may be hidden behind a facade of adequacy at work and superficial social adjustment.[7]

The paranoid patient may nurture his grudge for many years and attack when his name, or perhaps his very existence, has been forgotten by his victim. I recollect two such cases reported in the press, one about the time of World War II and the other one about 25 years ago. An orthopedist and a cardiologist who had been mistaken for the patient's psychiatrist were the victims. Podolski[8] believed that the purpose of a paranoid homicide is to discharge overwhelming rage. This reestablishes psychic homeostasis, helps to handle anxiety, and to gain a feeling if omnipotence. As murder by paranoids may be preceded by years of brooding, so also in malpractice suits the physician may be harassed and abused for years, particularly if the patient lost his case. This has been my experience with paranoid litigants.

Brancale[9] observed, in his rich experience, that the litigation and harassment give vent to the accumulated rage, and this may prevent bodily assault. This observation is probably correct, yet caution is recommended. The present climate of antiintellectualism, antielitism, and irrationality coupled with presentation of physicians, and particularly psychiatrists, as villains by the communication media, and such films as "*One Flew Over the Cuckoo's Nest,*" may abet pathological aggression and direct it against the physician. Murder of the physician is only one aspect of this aggression and release of rage. Feelings of helplessness, anxiety, rage, and frequently inferiority feed the paranoid's assaults.

Experts on violence recommend that the potential victim acknowledge and show fear in case of a threat and refuse to take the assailant's weapon, even if he offers it. This relieves his rage and feelings of helplessness.

In the case presented by Alliez and Savy,[2] paranoid phenomena started following an accident at work for which the patient had been awarded 100 percent compensation. Diffuse hypochondriacal complaints with depression are common following accidents. Expectation of reward certainly influences the patient's attitude in most of the cases, but the main fabric of posttraumatic mental states is infantile regression and the emergence of anxiety and rage among other factors.[10] It is therefore conceivable that exaggerated expectations of reward, and paranoid projections and elaborations, may be stimulated and released in predisposed individuals following trauma. It is my opinion that the examinations and reexaminations by many physicians, the depositions, a cold and businesslike approach by the examiners, and the whole adversary process surrounding the patient, aggravate the condition and increase the possibility of violence. Suicide following murder, as in the case of the murderer of Professor Pozzi, is well documented.[11] In some cases, the murderer may even demand capital punishment. Murder may follow suicidal preoccupations or there may be a combination of suicidal and homicidal fantasies.[12] A recent case of murder-suicide in New Jersey was reported in the press.[13] A disgruntled worker who lost his job and was not reinstated, shot himself after killing the company's founder and the two foremen who had testified against him in court. It is conceivable that a physician's testimony against a patient's claim in court may induce a similar outcome.

In some cases, the future murderer notifies his physician, friends, or minister that he may kill a specific person. This should not be taken lightly.[14] Unfortunately, a patient's warning frequently is not taken seriously.[12] A case in point is the well-known *Tarasoff* case in California. Tatiana Tarasoff, a student at the University of California at Berkeley, was killed by a young man who actually warned his psychotherapist of his intent. The psychotherapist notified the campus police, but the patient was not detained since "he looked normal." There is no preventive detention and patients committed to mental hospitals are discharged hastily through the "revolving door system." For this and other reasons, there is little protection against a paranoid litigant or a "persecuted persecutor." It is, therefore, an obligation to inform the potential victim of a threat to his life revealed by a patient to his physician, whether the prospective victim is a colleague or anyone else. This revelation of a patient's confidence should not be considered legally as a breach of confidentiality.

The case of A. B. initially presented in this paper belongs to the group of depressives with vague, continuous hypochrondriacal complaints with, or perhaps with only fleeting, paranoid symptoms. Murder and other crimes committed in depressive states were described by Woddis.[15] This, is my experience, is not uncommon. In the background of A. B.'s grudge, was the severe material and emotional deprivation of his early life, an abusive and rejecting father, and memories–still painful over four decades later–that he could not afford an ice cream cone in his childhood. A patient with a history of emotional deprivation and in need of support may interpret the lack of an immediate response by the physician as indifference and rejection. In fact, many suicides occur following such a perception of the physician's attitude. If the victim of A. B. had greeted him warmly in the waiting room, or had made some sign of recognition and concern, he still might be alive. Telling the patient that he would have only a short visit further increased A. B.'s feelings of rejection, indifference, and neglect. It is quite probable that the homicidal act was actually a transference reaction, the doctor paying with his life for the abuses of the patient's alcoholic father. Frazier[3] mentioned that some psychiatrists were victims of patients they had committed to a mental hospital and he advised to "do the patient the courtesy of a follow-up visit." It is, however, difficult and at times impossible for a busy practitioner to be available immediately and to make visits to distant hospitals. Patients, however, appreciate such an availability and this may save the life of (or at least a malpractice action against) an unsuspecting physician.

SUMMARY

Killing of physicians by their patients is relatively rare. Perhaps for this reason literature and research on the subject is scant. Two types of patients are likely to commit homicidal assaults on their physicians: the paranoid and the depressives with chronic complaints. The paranoids head the list by far. Urologists and proctologists, because of their dealing with areas of sexual significance, psychiatrists, and possibly orthopedists, are the main targets. It is suspected that legal involvement in a malpractice suit against the physician may absorb the paranoid patient's rage and thus deflect him from an assault on the physician. It is suggested to acknowledge and show fear in case of an assault by a paranoid patient, because this decreases the assailant's anxiety and feeling of helplessness. Ready availability to the patient will prevent not only many suicides, but also will prevent many malpractice suits and homicidal assaults.

REFERENCES

1. Dupré, M. (1918). Les medecins victimes de hypochondriaques persépersécuteurs meurtriers. *Bulletin de l'Académie de Médecine de Paris 80:* 78-84.
2. Alliez, J., & Savy, A. (1957). Deux observations de délirants meurtriers de medecins. *Annales Médico-Psycholoques, 114:*761-676.
3. Threat to kill psychiatrist should be taken seriously. *Clin Psych News, 5:*19, July, 1977.
4. Madden, D. J., & Lion, J. (1978). Treating the Violent Offender. *In violence: perspectives on murder and aggression* (Eds., Kutash, I. L., Kutash, S. B., & Schlesinger, L. B.) San Francisco: Josey Bass Inc.
5. Swanson, W. D., Bohnert, P. J., & Smith, J. A. (1970). *The paranoid.* Boston: Little, Brown.
6. *Malpractice Alert–Current Prescribing, 4:*27-28 (Dec) 1978.
7. Revitch, E. (1954). The problem of conjugal paranoia. *Dis Nerv Syst, 15:*271-277.
8. Podolsky, E. (1956). The paranoid murderer. *J Forensic Med, 3:*149-151.
9. Brancale, R. (1973). Personal Communication.
10. Roche, P. Q. (1960). The dynamics of neurosis following trauma. *Dis Nerv Syst, 21:*106-110.
11. West, D. J. (1966). *Murder followed by suicide.* Cambridge, MA: Harvard University Press.
12. Revitch, E., & Schlesinger, L. B. (1978). Murder: Evaluation, Classification and Prediction. In *Violence: perspectives on murder and aggression.* (Eds., Kutash, I. L., Kutash, S. B., & Schlesinger, L. B.) San Francisco, Josey Bass Inc.
13. Fired worker kills three, self at perfume plane. *The Star Ledger,* Sept. 12, 1978.
14. MacDonald, J. (1968). *Homicidal treats.* Springfield, IL: Charles C Thomas.
15. Woddis, G. (1957). Depression and crime. *Br J Delinquency, 8:*85-94.

Chapter 11

THE PROBLEM OF CONJUGAL PARANOIA

Of all the marital difficulties referred to the New Jersey State Diagnostic Center at Menlo Park by the Domestic Relations Courts, the paranoid state in one of the spouses presents the most difficult diagnostic and dispositional problem. In most cases, the paranoid state of the spouse had not been recognized previously to the examination at the Center, and it is usually the paranoid spouse who initiates a court action against the marital partner. Very often the plaintiff is able to win the sympathy of his or her family physician, the lawyer, neighbors and, of course, the immediate family, whose indignation has been mobilized and directed against the innocent marital partner. In one instance, where the couple was seen by a psychiatrist previous to the referral to the Center, the psychiatrist himself, after a rather cursory examination, considered the paranoid wife emotionally stable, and he gave the husband a lecture on morality and ethical conduct, thus dismissing the case (see Case 1).

I have not had the opportunity to make a statistical study of paranoid states in marital partners as the basis for marital difficulties, but I have an impression that it is by far a more frequent cause for discord than is generally recognized. The difficulty in diagnosis is due to the patient's lucidity, the frequently winning attitude in the interview situation, and the ability to present the facts in such a light that if one of the partners is suspected of being mentally ill, it may not be the patient, but his or her mate. It is wise therefore to examine the couple and not only one spouse. However, with extensive experience in this area, the psychiatrist is able to sense that he is dealing with a paranoid condi-

---

Source: Revitch, E. (1954). The problem of conjugal paranoia. *Diseases of the Nervous System, 15*:271-277.

tion, and if he devotes enough time to the examination, he may finally be rewarded with some gross misjudgment on the part of the patient which will confirm his earlier suspicion.

The difficulty in the disposition of these cases is due to the fact that the paranoiac may be productive, earn a living, support the family, or take care of the home and children. Commitment to a hospital, therefore, may be more disorganizing to the family unit than the constant squabbles between husband and wife. The result of shock therapy is disappointing. Psychotherapy is difficult to recommend, since the paranoid spouse feels that he or she should not be under treatment, but the mate, and therefore the psychiatric approach will usually be refused. Psychotherapy is not only rarely possible, but its results are uncertain. The problems of guardianship and custody of the children may be of great complexity and defy simple solutions since the patient may be able to conduct his or her business and be an adequate parent. Typical cases of the paranoid form of schizophrenia, or the paranoid form of involutional psychosis with severe personality disintegration, will be excluded from this study, since in these cases the problem of marital disorganization is the same as in any type of psychosis in one of the mates. In discussing the problem of conjugal paranoia, I refer to a paranoid state in one of the mates whose personality is well-integrated, whose delusional system concerns only the spouse, and is either rooted in some reality situation or concealed to such an extent that it may pass unnoticed.

CLINICAL PICTURE OF CONJUGAL PARANOIA

In practically all the cases under study, the first symptom of personality disorganization becomes obvious sometime after marriage, in many instances within the honeymoon period. Long before the appearance of the delusional system, the patient assumes critical attitudes, is fault-finding, humiliating and, in general, seems to do everything possible to degrade and demoralize the marital partner. This state of affairs produces marital discord, continuous bickering between spouses and unhappiness, which may precede by years the first evidence of delusional thinking. Sexual preoccupations may start immediately after marriage. The female is usually frigid and accuses her husband of being "hypersexed," a "pervert" or, to the contrary, impotent and disinterested. The male patient may show early potency disturbance, may request that his wife commit fellatio or submit to cunnilingus. In other instances, there may be a special interest in pornography or, to the contrary, extremely rigid, moralistic attitudes toward sex or a combination of both. As the condition progresses and takes root, some kind of separation, first of beds and then of bedrooms may take place. It is not unusual to see the mates sleeping apart for a number of years before the delusions become apparent.

After numerous squabbles, the patient may leave the spouse and go to live with parents or relatives, but even during periods of separation the actions and whereabouts of the mate are under continuous scrutiny. If the mate is satisfied with a separation, the patient may return and make attempts to resume the marital relationship, interfering in the mate's life. Yet, during the premarital courtship, the patient is frequently a satisfactory companion and often initiates the relationship. Almost always the paranoid spouse starts a whispering campaign against the mate, thus mobilizing the immediate family, acquaintances, and sometimes the community. It is needless to say that the indignation of the members of the immediate family against the innocent spouse is almost aroused by the patient. The patient is indiscreet in means of defamation, sometimes divulging family secrets or fabricating nonexistent situations. Thus, one of the patients wrote to the Draft Board that he would like a deferment for the sake of his wife, who conceived from him before they were married. This allegedly was done in an attempt to protect his wife from embarrassment but in reality, nothing embarrassed her more than this fact reported to the members of the Draft Board.

Situations may be created in which the mate will be seen in an unfavorable light by others. Thus, a female patient may provoke her husband into an argument, run out of the house and call neighbors and the police for help, claiming, often unjustly, that the husband had inflicted bodily injury to her. If the actions of the patient provoke a violent reaction in the mate, such as beating or defection of marital duties, the patient is able to point triumphantly to these facts, thus proving the unworthiness of the mate and justifying the complaint. The mate is always accused by the patient of being responsible for actions the patient himself initiated. For instance, in one case the wife accused the husband of not coming home and preferring to sleep in the store, thus neglecting marital duties. Further investigation, however, revealed that she locked the doors of the house, would not let the husband in, so that he was forced to sleep in his place of business (see Case 3).

Accusations of sexual perversion are frequent, particularly accusations of fellatio and cunnilingus or rectal intercourse. Yet, objective investigation always proves that it was the patient and not the mate (with a few exceptions) who initiated the less usual sexual practices. Accusing the mate of being mentally abnormal is frequent, and quite often during interviews with the patient he or she may ask to get psychiatric help for the spouse. Various acts with roots in reality will not only be perverted, but also fabricated. Thus, one patient brought to the office towels and toothpicks besmudged with lipstick, in order to prove "her husband's infidelity." She said it could not be her lipstick, since she stopped using it many years ago; yet, her lips were thickly colored with red while she was denying the use of lipstick (see Case 2). Not only the present reality, but also the past will be falsified and various occurrences and facts of the past involving the relationship of both spouses will be perverted. The delusional system may be present quite early or late and assume the form of jealousy and accusations of fidelity. The delusional system is centered around the mate and, if others are involved, they are involved only in their relationship to the mate. Thus, if a woman feels that all the other women in the neighborhood are prostitutes, she means that they have had affairs with her husband. Delusions such as the mate has intentions to kill the patient are less frequent and not related in a very convincing manner unless there are definite signs of a paranoid form of schizophrenia. The feeling attached to the delusional content is not jealousy, since jealousy implies love, but it consists in expression of contempt for the mate. In relating the delusions, the patient presents its content in such a way that the mate appears unworthy due to acts of infidelity. Thus, in one of my cases the paranoid husband stated that he would "forgive" his wife is she finally admitted to her "transgressions" (see Case 4).

Various means for apprehension of the mate during the commission of the "transgression" is devised to prove the spouses' immorality rather than actuated by pangs of jealousy. Strangers might be involved in the scheme to apprehend the "guilty" mate, and no discretion will be used. In one case, the husband called a physician and asked him to "investigate" his wife's genitals in order to determine whether she just had intercourse with someone else (see Case 4). In other words, when the patient goes out of the way to find out about the mate's "infidelity," it is not in the hope that the mate will be cleared, but with the hope that the suspicion will be supported by facts. In the interview the patient will give many "details" and "proofs" which sometimes have some basis in reality and therefore may mislead lawyers and judges.

Diagnostic Considerations

The question arises as to whether this condition deserves a special diagnostic category. Since in many instances the patient is able to function in areas other than conjugal relationship, it seems that a special diagnostic category is necessary for practical purposes. The condition presented here has the earmarks of what Kraepelin[1] described under the name of paranoia.

The name paranoia was previously used as a general term for "insanity with delusions." Kraepelin was the first to use it in the present sense. He defined paranoia as "an insidious development of a permanent and unshakeable delusional system, resulting from internal causes, which is accompanied by perfect perseveration of clear and orderly thinking, willing and acting." He remarked that in true paranoia there are no hallucinations and the patients "remain permanently sensible, clear and reasonable." Patient's delusions are usually of a persecutory and grandiose nature. The content of the persecutory delusions may be infidelity of the spouse coupled with pathological jealousy. In describing the delusions of jealousy, Kraepelin stated: "One is often in doubt how far real occurrences or delusional inventions are the foundation of what the patients say about the alleged suspicious observation, indeed, about the apparent admission of the husband." In addition to delusions, the patients may exhibit what Kraepelin referred to as "pseudo memories" (i.e., memory of events which never took place or which are a falsification of reality). As far as diagnosis is concerned, Kraepelin stressed that apart from general grounds of probability, paranoia should be suspected "if the patients adorn their narrative with very exact details, always increasing with repetition, when they produce their alleged observations a long time after the event."

In all the textbooks of psychiatry, true paranoia in the Kraepelinian sense is considered to be rare. In Kraepelin's statistics only one percent of admissions to mental hospitals could be classified as such. Yet, the admissions to mental hospitals do not give a clear-cut picture of the prevalence of the condition in the population, since many paranoiacs are able to work, to support themselves and their families and, in general, they may live through a lifetime without ever coming to the attention of a psychiatrist. The greater incidence of paranoia in the general population than reported, and the failure to diagnose the condition, was stressed in literature.[2]

Conjugal paranoia, being a true paranoia in the Kraepelinian sense, differs only in its more circumscribed and more specific content. As noted above, the psychotic nature of the condition may be difficult to recognize because of the "preservation of the clear and orderly thinking, willing, and acting." Like in Kraepelin's description of paranoia, there are pseudo-memories, adornment of the narrative with details, and the delusional content may have some foundation in reality so that "one is often in doubt how far real occurrences or delusional inventions are the foundation of what the patients say about the alleged suspicious observation." Yet, the diagnostic problem may be more complex if the clear delusional system has not been formed as yet, and the condition is chiefly characterized by the patient's contemptuous, destructive, demanding, fault-finding and critical attitudes toward the mate. In cases of this type, there is no manifestation which could be clearly qualified as psychotic. The patient may be considered just "jealous," or "mean," but since neither his meanness nor jealousy appear bizarre, the whole affair may be dismissed as incompatibility between spouses.

The projective techniques frequently show confusion in sexual identification, suspiciousness, evasiveness, self-destructive tendencies, dependency, poor self-concept and poor controls. They are frequently helpful in determining which of the spouses is the sicker; however, in my experience, several reports by three well trained and experienced psychologists failed to reveal serious personality disintegration in spite of the presence of delusional thinking with a rather bizarre content. This can probably be explained by a rather good preservation of the personality structure and intellectual controls in many cases of paranoia. An unhurried, thorough clinical examination of the patient and the spouse by the same psychiatrist remains, in my opinion, the most accurate tool in the diagnosis of conjugal paranoia.

A question arises as to whether paranoia and paranoid schizophrenia are two different entities or different degrees of the same condition? Even Kraepelin recognized that some of his true paranoics later on developed symptoms of the paranoid form of schizophrenia. He felt, however, that if properly diagnosed, paranoia and the paranoid form of dementia praecox presented two separate entities; that is, true paranoia would not develop into the paranoid form of dementia praecox.

CASE HISTORIES

Case 1

Mrs. C., a 31-year-old woman, mother of two children, married for approximately ten years, filed a complaint of inadequate support and requested inquiry into her marital status. The early part of the marital history was not remarkable, except that Mrs. C. had some difficulties with other women while following her husband to various Army camps during his service. After discharge from the service, the couple moved close to Mr. C's family. Mr. C., dominated, to some extent by his family, entered into a disadvantageous business venture with his brother.

Real difficulties started seven years after marriage, following the birth of a second child. Mrs. C. decided, at first, to sleep apart from her husband. This, however, was interrupted off and on by a week or so of a honeymoon relationship, but then again Mrs. C. slept apart in a different room, and threatened to leave the house. She became more and more irritable and on many occasions was seen upset and crying. The husband's attempt to resume a friendly relationship usually failed, and once when he asked if she wanted him to bring her a cup of coffee, she answered, "I wouldn't be surprised if you put poison in this coffee."

Mrs. C. started complaining to neighbors about her husband abusing and mistreating her. Her family physician was so impressed by her "woes" that he helped her contact a lawyer. When another physician, suspecting a mental disorder, sent the couple to a psychiatrist, the latter, after a short interview, declared that Mrs. C. "was of sound mind" and told the husband to treat his wife with more consideration. Meanwhile, Mrs. C. spread news that she was in love with a man in the neighborhood, and she claimed that she went out with this man and his family to the seashore since they were planning to be married. She talked about it without reserve to strangers and to her husband, who never saw his wife and the neighbor together, but nevertheless believed the story.

Mrs. C. was attractively attired and obviously tried to impress during the interview. Her speech was well-connected. She seemed to be lucid, cultured, intelligent, and somewhat sophisticated. Since she was interviewed before her husband, her account gave the impression that I was dealing with a gifted woman who was just tired of her inadequate and insecure husband and of the domination of his immediate family. However, here and there, during the interview, she made sly remarks about her husband's intentions which put me on guard. In the beginning, I could find nothing but her emphasis on her husband's peculiar sexual preferences (husband later admitted that it was true), such as shaving her pubic hair, liking to bathe her, and occasionally insisting on cunnilingus and fellatio. Then she reported that during one of their reconciliations he took her to a restaurant in New York where he acted "like a big shot" to impress her. She intimated that this invitation had some hidden meaning. She also reported that she found matches from a restaurant, again intimating that her husband, for some reason, spent his time away from home.

Mrs. C. was able to gain the sympathy of people she was in contact with, yet her behavior was inconsistent. For instance, she related even to strangers the story of being in love with another man, at the same time filing a complaint of nonsupport against her husband. When this complaint was investigated, it was found to be unfounded. The story of having gone out with another man was also unfounded and was probably what Kraepelin considered a "pseudo-memory." Later on, further investigation showed that about a year or so ago the husband was brought home by a rescue squad after an automobile accident. Mrs. C. felt at the time, that her husband was just faking; therefore, she called the police station to find out whether there really had been an accident. In this case no bizarre delusional material was elicited, but the patient expressed her delusional thinking by various intimations and remarks, seeing in simple events some kind of a hidden meaning.

Case 2

Mr. and Mrs. D. were referred because of marital difficulties and Mrs. D.'s complaints of her husband's infidelity. At the time of the examination, the husband was 51 years old, the wife 38 years old. Mr. D. was married previously and divorced his first wife after fourteen years due to poor relations between them. It was Mrs. D.'s first marriage, and she met Mr. D. when she was only 25 years old. The couple had been married for ten years at the time of the examination. Shortly after marriage, Mrs. D. became suspicious of her husband and on many occasions she left him, going to her mother's home and then coming back unexpectedly. This led to several short separations.

A few months prior to the interview, Mrs. D.'s behavior became very unreasonable. She claimed that another woman was coming to the house. She allegedly found nail polish on the garage door and lipstick on toothpicks and towels. She destroyed furniture and, on one occasion, she shot the house with a BB gun. Since she destroyed his furniture, Mr. D. was forced to put another lock on the door so that she could not get in. In the office during the interview, Mrs. D. was well-dressed, neatly groomed, friendly–making a nice impression. She talked fluently, was able to give biographical data in good chronological order. She was well-oriented and in good contact with her surroundings.

However, it became obvious that she acted under the influence of paranoid delusions. She was very circumstantial, and gave many details to illustrate her point. She produced towels and toothpicks with lipstick "to prove that another woman was coming to her house." She claimed it could not be her lipstick, since she had stopped using it when she discovered that someone else was coming to her house. She claimed that she came back home unexpectedly to check on her husband and, when she came in, he gave her a cold greeting thus hurting her feelings. She also stopped having sexual relations with him, because she did not want to "share him with another woman." To substantiate her complaints, she stated that once she found a smudge of lipstick on the door of the bathroom and this, she thought, was done deliberately by the other woman in order to irritate her. On one occasion, she also found a "hair of another woman" on the visor of her husband's car. Later on, talking to the psychologist during administration of the psychological tests, she told him that this "was a vaginal hair." Therefore she pulled a hair out of her pubic area and put it on the visor to "show the woman that she was still around."

In talking about the beginning of her marriage, Mrs. D. reported that girls greeted her husband, "Hello Rob" and asked him "if he will be there," thus implying that even then, 10 years ago, he already was unfaithful to her. She also accused him of being oversexed to the point that her vagina became sore, and that he attempted to practice abnormal sex relations with her.

In this case, there are a great deal of pseudo-memories and paranoid delusions with erotic content. In spite of the fact that Mrs. D. was extremely disorganized, as far as her behavior and thinking are concerned, she may impress one during a casual conversation as an intelligent, interesting and charming woman. The towels and toothpicks with lipstick which she produced as "evidence" should not mislead, since it is obvious the lipstick was from her own lips (in spite of her statement that she stopped using lipstick, yet in the office, her lips were thickly covered with it).

Case 3

Mr. and Mrs. E. were referred because of marital discord. At the time of the examination, the husband was 40 years old, the wife 34. When examined, the couple had been married ten years. Difficulties started right after marriage. At first, Mrs. E. felt that three sexual relations a week was abnormal. She forced her husband to reduce to once a week. Later on, she felt that this was also abnormal and very frequently she refused relations, stating that she had her period. Several years before, Mr. E. had started his own business, but Mrs. E. did everything to ruin it. She started accusing him of having sexual relations with a policeman's wife; she made scenes at home; at times she did not let him into the house and he had to sleep on the floor at his place of business. Mrs. E. complained to her minister, to her lawyer, and to the policeman that her husband was a sex pervert, and she accused most of the women in the neighborhood of being prostitutes. One morning, when her husband went to the post office and returned in twenty minutes, she accused him of having had intercourse with a girl who lived down the street. She also felt people were not neighborly, because she came from the South.

In the interview, Mrs. E. was pleasant, cooperative and talkative. Listening to her one could picture her husband as a stupid, bragging, and brutal individual in need of psychiatric care. Her account sounded plausible until she reported, although without conviction, that her husband threatened to kill her. She accused him of situations for which she herself was responsible. Thus, she blamed her husband for sleeping in the store instead of coming home, when in reality she herself barred his entrance. She also accused him of being a sex pervert who forced her to commit fellatio. She claimed that he was going with other women and she made disparaging remarks about his claims of being a business man. In general, she did everything to put him in a bad light.

Case 4

Mr. G., a 55-year-old male who immigrated to the United States from Germany in 1924, filed a complaint in the Domestic Relations Court charging his wife with being indifferent and quarrelsome. The wife, 47 years old, is the mother of two children born to the couple in 1942 and 1944. At the time of the examination the couple had been married about 19 years. In 1925, Mrs. G. was forcibly married (by her parents) to an elderly man, but she soon left him and when the latter died, she struck up an acquaintance with Mr. G. who was a neighbor in the same rooming house.

Difficulties between both spouses started almost immediately after marriage. There was constant bickering, fights, and mutual accusations. Mr. G. was described by his wife as a very dependent, childish individual, subject to temper tantrums during which he occasionally broke dishes and stamped his feet. At the same time, he attempted to assume the attitude of the "lord" of the family, demanding obedience and respect from his wife, yet relying on her in business and management of home affairs. Mr. G. frequently had to take a "rest" and "relax" while his wife labored with the children and in the store. An incident was described when, shortly after marriage, he told her that his friends meant more to him than she did. He frequently left her alone and went to New York to visit these friends. Very early after marriage he beat her. The beatings were provoked, he said, by arguments concerning money. On one occasion, he threw his wife to the floor and commanded that she crawl before him, which she refused to do. On many occasions, he would come home in a bad mood, look for dust on the walls and dirt in the corners, accusing his wife of being untidy.

About 10 years before this examination, Mr. G. requested that they sleep in twin beds. For the past six years, they have had no sex at all. He was never too potent and never, throughout the marriage, have they had relations more than once a month. Approximately eight to nine months before the examination, Mr. G. started accusing his wife of going out with other men. At approximately that time, Mrs. G. suffered a fractured arm and, when she went to the doctor for treatment, Mr. G. questioned her inquisitively about the time she spent outside of the home. Each time she was a little late coming home, or talked to a customer in the store, he felt that she was having an affair with someone. Once when she came back from the doctor's office, he followed her upstairs and asked her who had brought her home. Then he looked around the rooms, opened the closets, and finally said, "It is funny that no one is here," thus implying that he suspected his wife of coming home with somebody else. On one occasion, when she came home with an attack of headache and lay down, he looked at her inquisitively, and said she looked poorly, and called a doctor to examine her. When the doctor arrived, he asked him to examine her genitals, since he suspected that she had been out with a man and therefore had a headache. When the children were born he was cold and reserved, but within the past year or so he became more attentive to them, in an effort to alienate them from their mother.

In the interview, Mr. G. was well-dressed, courteous and gentlemanly. He spoke slowly and deliberately about his marriage. He reported that it was very hard to satisfy his wife, that she wanted him to do everything her way but, in reality, this did not trouble him as much as her desire to break up the marriage. He accused her of being immoral with other men, and he said that he would forgive her if she would just admit her immorality.

He reported that once, coming back from town, she left the car outside. When he checked the car, he saw the windows were "steamed up." When asked what this meant to him, he answered that it looked "as if more than one person had been in the car breathing heavily, as usually happens during sexual intercourse." He added, "In my opinion there shouldn't be any secrets in marriage." When asked whether he would like to break up the marriage, he answered emphatically, "No."

As in other cases of conjugal paranoia, the projective tests did not reveal grave personality disintegration, in spite of the fact that the routine mental examination elicited definite delusions of a paranoid nature. In this case, the paranoid delusions were preceded by 18 years of hostile, humiliating and destructive attitudes, without any other evidence of psychotic thinking. Mr. G. had been productive, able to manage a store, although relying largely on his wife. During the interview, he constantly projected his own thoughts on his wife and related the story in such a way that she, rather than he, would have been suspected of paranoia had he not revealed frank delusional material.

Etiological Considerations

A question arises as to whether the patients under study would have developed paranoia in some other form if they remained single? Liber[3] reported six patients with mild depression and psychosomatic symptoms which, in his opinion, were entirely due to marital conflicts. He believed that marital conflicts are, on the whole, important contributory factors to some mental illness. Freud[4] reported the case of a young man who developed episodes of delusions of jealousy, the object of which was his wife, and which always appeared on the day following the act of intercourse. Since Freud believed that paranoia was a defense against homosexuality, he felt that in this particular case, "after every satiation of the heterosexual libido, the homosexual component, likewise stimulated by the act, forced for itself an outlet in the attack of jealousy." Whether in this case the episodes of paranoid jealousy were due to stimulated homosexuality or to other causes, the fact remains that paranoid explosions were connected with sexual activity of the patient.

The projective tests in this study indicate that these patients are insecure, weak, dependent, suspicious personalities with confusion in sexual identification. Clinical investigation frequently reveals sexual preoccupations, frigidity, and low potency. In addition, one of my female patients revealed that she always preferred to be a man, and another female patient bore the male name of Lester, given to her by her parents who had been greatly disappointed by not having a boy. Furthermore, in a large number of cases, spouses use separate beds, and later on rooms, for a number of years preceding the onset of delusions. Thus, the studies conducted here seem to indicate that homosexual awareness or, at least some degree of confusion in sexual identification, is quite common. This seems to support Freud's views on homosexuality in the genesis of paranoia. The extremely hostile and humiliating attitudes toward the spouse are probably a projection of the patient's hostility toward himself. Since the patients feel weak, insecure and, in many instances, relies on the spouse for the management of their affairs, I believe that the humiliating and superior attitudes toward the spouse are also a reaction formation to these dependent needs and to low concept of one's self. Mr. G. (in Case 4) for instance ordered his wife to crawl before him, and yet, playing the role of a "lord," he relied on her to manage his business, and was quite upset when she stopped helping him.

I have not had the opportunity to follow patients who separated from their spouses, but since conjugal relations seem to be the precipitating cause of their attitudes and delusions, I believe that at least, in some cases, great improvement may be obtained. Conjugal relations, by which I mean not only sexual intercourse, but everything that are part of the responsibilities of a spouse, and possibly parent, induce in the patient a general feeling of inadequacy. Such individuals cope by utilizing the defense mechanisms of projection and reaction formation.

SUMMARY

An attempt is made to demonstrate a specific type of paranoia, with delusions and pathological attitudes directed against the marital partner. The pathological attitudes characterized by humiliating and destructive acts against the spouse may precede, by many years, the outbreak of frank paranoid delusions. The patient always preserves good contact with the environment and is able to conduct his or her affairs. The paranoiac may be able to veil projections so skillfully that not the patient, but the spouse, may be considered either abnormal, or may become the target of indignation of the patient's immediate family, neighbors, and so forth.

Projective techniques do not always elicit the gravity of the clinical condition. But testing is valuable in the evaluation of the personality structure of the patient and, in cases where both spouses are under suspicion, testing may indicate which one is the sicker. The best diagnostic tool, however, is an unhurried and careful interview of both spouses by the same psychiatrist. The problem of disposition is also extremely difficult, defying simple solutions, due to the apparent lucidity and productive capacity of the patient. The patients who develop conjugal paranoia are inadequate and weak individuals, with confusion in sexual identification. Homosexual conflicts and a general feeling of inadequacy, aggravated by the conjugal relationship, seems to be the most important factors in he genesis of conjugal paranoia. Four representative cases were reported.

REFERENCES

1. Kraepelin, E. (1921). *Manic-depressive insanity and paranoia*. Edinburgh: E. and S. Livingstone.
2. Bonner, H. (1951). The problem of diagnosis in paranoid disorders. *Am. J. of Psychiat., 107*:677-683.
3. Liber, B. (1950). Elusive mental cases: Marital conflicts. *N.Y. State J. Med., 50*:2287-89.
4. Freud, S. (1922). Certain neurotic mechanisms in jealousy, paranoia and homosexuality. *Collected Papers, Vol. II.* (1948). London: The Hogarth Press.

Chapter 12

THE PARANOID MARITAL PARTNER: COUNSELOR'S CLIENT, PSYCHIATRIST'S PROBLEM

In 1890, approximately once divorce was granted in the United States for every sixteen marriages performed. Recognizing the ever-increasing population in our country today, it is still astounding to realize that in 1947 the number of successful litigants in the divorce courts equaled nearly one-third the number of couples entering into the bonds of matrimony, with the future holding little hope of any immediate reduction in the percentage of ill-fated marriages. It is not a wonder then that, among others concerned, the legal profession has become alarmed at this trend and has taken action to study the problem and to arrest the advancing tide of broken homes.[1]

In many cases of disrupted marital life, mental derangements in one or both of the marital partners may be the basis for their difficulties. The senior author has been attracted by the prevalence of a specific type of psychosis unfavorably affecting marital relations. This condition is difficult to recognize, and because it has all the appearances of normalcy, may easily mislead both the bench and the bar.[2] It is our object to illustrate to the lawyer the various social and legal problems that this condition may entail.

Source: Revitch, E. & Hayden, J. W. (1955). The paranoid marital partner: Counselor's client, psychiatrist's problem. *Rutgers Law Review, 9*:512-527.

A CLINICAL STUDY OF CONJUGAL PARANOIA

The word paranoia was previously used as a general term for insanity with delusions.[3] Emil Kraepelin, the great systematizer for psychiatric conditions[4] was the first to use paranoia in the present sense. He defined it as "an insidious development of a permanent and unshakeable delusional system, resulting from internal causes, which is accompanied by perfect preservation of clear and orderly thinking, willing and acting." He remarked that in true paranoia there is no hallucinations,[5] and that ". . . the patients remain permanently sensible, clear and reasonable." The delusions which characterize this condition are usually of a persecutory or grandiose nature. The content of persecutory delusions may be infidelity of the spouse coupled with pathological jealousy. In addition to the delusions, the patient exhibits what Kraepelin refers to as "pseudo-memories," i.e. memory of events which have never taken place. The "pseudo-memories may be so much within the realm of possibility that it is difficult to differentiate them from the truth.

In all the textbooks of psychiatry, true paranoia in the Kraepelin sense is considered to be rare. By Kraepelin's statistics, one percent of admissions to mental hospitals could be classified as such. Yet, the admissions to mental hospitals do not give a clear-cut picture of the prevalence of the condition in the population, as many paranoics are able to work, to support themselves and their families and, in general, may live through a lifetime without ever coming to the attention of a psychiatrist.[6]

There are also other mental conditions where paranoid delusions are prominent in the symptomatology. These include the paranoid form of schizophrenia, involutional psychosis, some senile dementiae, and so forth. However, individuals with these conditions are overtly psychotic and present no serious difficulty in diagnosis and disposition, as they usually result in admission to a mental hospital.

Conjugal paranoia is a true paranoia in the Kraepelinian sense, but here the delusional system concerns only marital relations and the patient is able to function in other life situations. The delusions are either rooted in some reality situation or concealed to such an extent that they may pass unnoticed. The difficulty in diagnosis is due to the patient's apparent lucidity, the frequent winning attitude in the interview situation, and the ability to present the facts in such a way that if one of the partners is suspected of being mentally ill, it may not be the patient, but his or her mate.

In practically all the cases under study, the first symptom of personality disorganization becomes obvious sometime after marriage, in many instances within the honeymoon period. Long before the appearance of the delusional system, the patient assumes critical attitudes, is faultfinding, humiliating, and seems to do everything possible to degrade and demoralize the marital partner. During this period, diagnosis is most difficult as there is not a manifestation which could be clearly qualified as psychotic. The patient may be considered just "jealous," or "mean," and the whole affair dismissed as incompatibility between spouses. The delusional system, when it appears, often assumes the form of jealously and accusations of infidelity.

In a typical situation, the paranoid marital partner will initiate court action against the spouse. It may be a complaint of nonsupport, infidelity, or abuse. Investigation of the complaint may or may not substantiate the complainant's statements. In the latter case, the procedure is simplified, as a suspicion of mental derangement should immediately arise. In the former case, a deeper investigation will prove that the defendant's actions were provoked by the complainant. Thus for instance, the complainant may provoke an argument and then run out of the house calling neighbors or police, exaggerating the defendant's alleged abuse. In this situation, the pathological reaction of the complainant is obscured by a demonstrable fact.

The patient will frequently bring many details into the discussion, sometimes pertaining to events or alleged events of the past. He will also bring various "proofs" to the attorney or the court in order to present his case. An example of this is the case of Mrs. A., who complained of her husband's infidelity (see Case 1 in the Appendix).

Because the delusions are so well-systematized, and sometimes have a factual basis, the lawyer, judge, immediate family and the family physician may be won over by the paranoid mate. Furthermore, due to the lucidity of the plaintiff, the grave diagnosis and prognosis given by a psychiatrist may leave the lawyer incredulous and make him seek the opinion of another expert. Examples of this are seen in Cases 2 and 3, where a paranoid condition existed in one of the marital partners, yet where a lawyer, doctors, and in one instance a psychiatrist at first failed to recognize it (see Cases 2 and 3 in the Appendix).

Almost always then, the paranoid spouse starts a whispering campaign against the mate, thus mobilizing the immediate family, acquaintances, and sometimes the community (see Case 4 in the Appendix). At times the accusations of the paranoid spouse, particularly if it is the wife, may be substantiated in the eyes of others by actions of the husband. For instances, he is accused of slapping his wife. Indeed, he did slap her, but the slapping was provoked by constant nagging, accusations, and spying. Perhaps the tension at home, the incomprehensible behavior of the wife keeps him away, and occasionally he may be found in the company of another woman. The paranoid mate may also be a major factor in creating the situation of which he or she complains, but because of the peculiarities of his or her reasoning, has dismissed the role he or she played in creating such situations (see Case 5 in the Appendix).

Accusations of sexual perversion are frequent, particularly accusations of *fellatio and cunnilingus* or rectal intercourse. Yet, objective investigation always proves that it was the patient and not the mate (with a few exceptions), who initiated the less usual sexual practices. Accusing the mate of being mentally abnormal is frequent, and quite often during interviews with the patient he or she may ask to get psychiatric help for the spouse. Various acts with roots in reality will be not only distorted, but also fabricated.

In experience with these cases, more women than men have shown paranoid behavior in the marital situation. Kraepelin stated that 70 percent of his paranoics were males, but the erotic delusions were more frequent in women. As to the cause of paranoia and paranoid conditions, Freud's[7] theory that paranoia is a defense against latent homosexuality seems to be the most popular in the United States. Kraepelin[8] and Meyer,[9] however, felt that paranoid delusions were a defense measure against disappointments in life. Adler's[10] views were quite similar and, in his opinion, some people could develop paranoia merely by facing life's difficulties. It should be noted that the patients who develop conjugal paranoia are inadequate and emotionally weak individuals with confusion in sexual identification. Homosexual conflicts and a general feeling of inadequacy, aggravated by the conjugal relationship, seem to be the most important factors in the genesis of conjugal paranoia.

In brief, then, this is the problem we have outlined which confronts the unwitting lawyer: other than the delusions with which he or she is suffering, and which generally cannot be detected and recognized as such by the untrained eye, the paranoid litigant generally presents a picture of a perfect, mentally balanced and rational individual. Some of the facts stated by the paranoic may be substantiated, but the meanings and conclusions which this person derives from these acts, and on which he or she bases the cause of action are completely erroneous.[11] Again, because of otherwise rational behavior, he or she will be able to convince the unsuspecting attorney, or perhaps the court, of the validity of his or her accusations.

RECOGNIZING THE PARANOID LITIGANT

The problem described above may affect the lawyer in several ways. He or she may have as his or her client the paranoid-plaintiff spouse who presents an apparently good cause of action. Without careful investigation on the part of the attorney, and close scrutiny of his own client, the result may be costly, wasteful, and embarrassing. On the other hand, the lawyer may be faced with the problem of defending an innocent spouse against the accusations and action of the paranoid mate. Unless she has some comprehension of what the true situation is, she may be unable to convince anyone that her client is really the innocent party. This is not to mention, in addition, the imposition on our courts.

In the converse situations (i.e., that of defending the paranoid spouse against court action, or seeking a divorce, and so forth., for his client from the paranoid mate), the lawyer who recognizes this condition may be able to play the role of humanitarian as well as legal counsel. A full explanation of the condition to the healthy spouse may help in keeping the couple together, as it gives the healthy partner a different perspective and may lead to some readjustment of the situation. Couples have lived together for years, as long as the healthy partner realized that his spouse was ill. Furthermore, even in paranoia, there may be periods of congenial behavior. Psychotherapy or shock therapy will not effect a "cure," but psychiatric help may be beneficial in alleviating, to some extent, the tense marital relationship. Hospitalization in these cases is generally not the answer; however, divorce is by no means the only solution to the situation.

The reason for the difficulty in recognizing the paranoid condition is apparent. In spite of the paranoia, the individual may function socially, may still be a rather adequate parent, and frequently is the sole support of the family. The psychotic material is generally scattered and concealed and will be brought up to the surface only with skillful examination. Of course, when the case is presented in written form, all the material indicating the psychotic process is concentrated in such a way that the psychotic nature of the patient becomes very evident. However, this does not occur except as a result of a full psychiatric examination. There are certain characteristics, some of which we have illustrated, which will aid both the lawyer and the court in recognizing this condition when it initially appears before them.

Kraepelin[12] stresses that apart from general grounds of probability, the diagnosis of paranoia should be suspected "if the patients adorn their narrative with very exact details, always increasing with repetition, when they produce their alleged observations a long time after the event." These details, from the lawyer's point of view, may not be necessary at all and are uncalled for by him in his interview or questioning. But to the paranoic, they are essential both to convince the attorney of the validity of his statements, and perhaps as a form of self-reassurance.

Another tendency of the paranoic which will manifest itself in the lawyer's office is to produce "evidence" in support of his or her story which, to even the inexperienced, will appear irrelevant, and on closer examination may even prove false. In one of the recent cases a husband, who later was diagnosed as paranoid, appeared at an interview and produced pictures which he had had taken of clothes lying outside his house on a doorstep (allegedly they were his and had been thrown there by his wife in an outburst of temper), of a cow's skull and horn adorning his wife's favorite wall, and of himself, half stripped, with several bruises on his back and chest (allegedly placed there by his wife during one of their arguments). An investigation led to the conclusion that the clothes had been placed on the doorstep, and the bruises applied with paint, by the patient himself for the benefit of the photographs. It should be noted that these people are not conscious of their lies or exaggerations. They may know that they falsified a picture, or taunted the other person into beating them, but this has been discarded in their minds, and they become convinced that they actually suffered in the manner they described.

Frequent sexual accusations of a distorted nature against the other partner are perhaps the most common characteristic of persons afflicted with conjugal paranoia. As illustrated by the earlier cases, they will claim that the partner is sexually abnormal, describing specific activities or attitudes to emphasize this, when in truth an entirely opposite situation exists. Alternatively, the paranoic actually desires or causes the sexual situation for which the mate is accused. Another characteristically paranoid reaction is the willingness to relate these activities to anyone who is interested. The paranoid person is inconsiderate and will divulge family secrets, whether true or false, without hesitation.

There is a similar prevalence of mental accusations in the paranoid's story, and as stated before, he will hasten to align a multitude of irrelevant "facts" to convince his audience of the abnormality of the other person. Instead of forthright accusations, however, the charge may take on a cloak of concealment, i.e., that of perverting or inverting the facts to make the listener merely suspect the opposite partner of being abnormal. There is also a strong tendency on the part of the paranoic to exaggerate his or her own attributes, alleged faults of the mate, and his or her own resultant suffering. The paranoic will also be insulting, particularly so to his marital partner. The manifestation of this tendency will vary, however, according to the individual's social level and, in some cases, may be difficult for an outsider to detect.

PROBLEMS OF THE ATTORNEY FOR THE PARANOIC: PLAINTIFF AND DEFENDANT

Once an attorney recognizes or suspects this condition in his or her client, it is simple enough to deal with the problem. As some of our juvenile and domestic relations courts are now doing, referral of both parties for a psychiatric examination may prove invaluable in clearing the facts and settling the matter expediently.[13] A tactful lawyer should find no great problem in convincing a plaintiff-client who is under suspicion of paranoia that were the client and the mate both examined by a psychiatrist, an alternate solution to the proposed legal action might be found for their difficulties. There would, of course, be no basis for a lawyer to indicate to such a client that he or she was under such suspicion, and the entire situation must be handled with care. A lawyer, or for that matter any lay person, should never attempt to make such a diagnosis himself; this is the psychiatrist's field. In fact, the need for informal professional contact between the lawyer and a psychiatrist, prior to any formal contact or recommendation for examination to the parties, is apparent.

On the other hand, focusing only on the legal problems and not on the counseling possibilities noted above, if the suspected paranoic client is a defendant in the action, he or she may very glad to grasp at any defense available. Full insanity at the time of the alleged act, constituting grounds for divorce, is a defense to the action in New Jersey. However, conjugal paranoia is not, it would seem to be the type of insanity which falls within this defense, for the defendant must be insane generally and not suffering merely from delusions. In *Youmans v Youmans*,[14] the wife, without grounds, repeatedly accused her husband of infidelity, yet offered no proof or valid reasons to substantiate this, later deserting him. The court held that the wife, in a divorce action brought by her husband, must prove full insanity at the time she committed the acts complained of, if she relies on this as a defense. In the absence of this showing, there will be granted an absolute divorce to the husband. The court noted that the wife's actions, as shown even in the evidence introduced by her husband, indicated delusions and possible partial insanity. This court also cited the earlier case of *Smith v. Smith*,[15] wherein the husband suffered delusions that his wife continually committed incest with their son, and consequently pursued an erratic course of action, accusing her without real cause, spying on and at times striking her, and in general making her fear for her life. In granting a separation, the court also noted that the husband did not appear entirely sane. Thus, it would seem that conjugal paranoia *per se*, is not a defense to a divorce action in New Jersey. However, it may well be introduced in an attempt to explain away the paranoic-defendant's behavior, and thus encourage the court and the parties to reexamine marriage counseling possibilities.

PROBLEMS WHEN THE ADVERSARY IS THE PARANOIC: DEFENDANT AND PLAINTIFF

Another problem arises for the attorney when he is defending the sane partner against his or her paranoic spouse, and the case is proceeding to litigation. Even though the lawyer may recognize a paranoic condition in the accuser, and firmly believes in the lack of fault or guilt in his or her own client, how can the lawyer convince the court? How can the attorney convince those who might aid the psychotic plaintiff of the validity of his suspicions and thus avoid or defeat the impending litigation?

Whether in court or at a pretrial conference, the lawyer should attempt to confront both spouses with the same complained facts or episodes. As we have seen before, the situations which the paranoic describes may be rooted in reality, but when he or she interprets and relates them as facts, they are highly exaggerated so that false conclusions may be drawn. Compare the testimony of the two parties. The paranoic may have given a good impression and convinced his or her audience of the story. A comparison of the sane and insane persons and their testimony will illustrate to listeners, by the very unreasonableness and extremeness of one side, the paranoid condition of the accuser. It is well to note, however, that paranoics firmly believe in what they say. Though they understand and would respect an oath for what it means, they in fact believe themselves to be telling the truth. They have no fear of sanctions imposed for false or exaggerated statements relating to their marital affairs. A paranoic may expose himself on the witness chair by the very nature of his statements, but he will not expose himself by any mannerisms reflective of consciousness of guilt.[16]

Thus, the attorney should attempt to elicit a statement of an unreasonable or extreme nature, which will be seen as obviously delusional in character. If the accuser shows a strong inference of suffering from delusions, the opposing attorney has rebutted the testimony and perhaps stalemated the action. At least, he would have logical grounds to counterclaim, placing the mental condition of the plaintiff into controversy, and to request a psychiatric examination of the party before proceeding.[17]

Challenging a suspected paranoic's statement, in view of the fact that positive proof means little in a delusion, may appear futile. However, if practiced skillfully, this can prove rewarding. The paranoic cannot be "talked out of" even a deliberate lie, void of any real factual basis, for his mind has forgotten that it is a lie, and he is firmly convinced of its truth. On the other hand, he or she may become responsive to the challenge, and seeing that his statement is in doubt, may attempt to convince his listeners. If he or she can be kept talking enough, it is more than likely he will either contradict himself or exaggerate into the realm of absurdity the situation he is describing. Again, his statements taken separately may all be logical and often partially substantiated, but when combined and summarized, the context will very likely illustrate the unreasonableness of his or her testimony and absence of mental balance, as it pertains to the marital relationship, beneath his disguise of apparent lucidity and rationality.

If the defendant lawyer's suspicion as to the mental capacity of the plaintiff are aroused prior to trial, he may also want to retain a psychiatrist to observe the plaintiff, listen to the testimony during the trial, and give his or her expert advice. If the opinion of the psychiatrist bears out the attorney's suspicion, it may be possible to attack the credibility of the plaintiff by introducing the expert testimony. More likely, however, the psychiatrist will be unable to come to a conclusion as to the delusional nature of the plaintiff's statements without a more thorough examination. Even if the result of the expert testimony is merely to the effect that the plaintiff's statements seem incredible, followed by a recommendation that a psychiatric examination should take place, the court may be influenced to do so. Precisely, this problem has been described in advancing the possibility of using "testimonial witnesses," i.e., psychiatric advice to the trial court concerning the capacity of certain witnesses to testify, based on an examination of the witnesses by a psychiatrist subsequent to their testimony.[18] *Caveat*, however, as stated in the aforementioned article, for possible unsettled legal problems and new procedural problems which inevitably arise when opening new fields of court procedure, particularly from a proposal of this scope and effect. Such problems are beyond the scope of this article, and are neither proposed nor discussed.

If the court finds that the allegations in the complaint are fallacious, the action will be dismissed and the parties left to solve their marital difficulties as best they can. Even, however, if the court finds, in addition, that the plaintiff-spouse is paranoic, under our present statutes,[19] this, *per se*, will not give the vindicated spouse the grounds for his or her own divorce action. Unless the defendant has other grounds on which he or she has based a counterclaim in the original action, the most that can be hoped for is, again, a dismissal. As yet, insanity is not grounds for divorce in New Jersey, and even it if were, it is doubtful if conjugal paranoia would fall within the type of insanity necessary to comprise such a ground. This is true by virtue of the same reasons as those for the conclusion stated above, that conjugal paranoia probably does not come within the types of insanity, which are a defense to the action.

The remaining situation, i.e., that of representing the sane plaintiff-spouse against the paranoic mate, poses no novel legal problem but rather, as mentioned above, presents the attorney who recognizes the situation with an opportunity to counsel the parties. The sane plaintiff will probably have good grounds for the action, and the defendant no legal defense, but if this client can be made to understand why his or her spouse acted in the manner that he or she did, the desire for divorce or separation may be eliminated and the plaintiff may seek instead to reconstruct his or her crumbling castle.

APPENDIX

Case histories of the paranoid patients described here and pertinent to the preceding article are taken from the files of Doctor Eugene Revitch at the State Diagnostic Center, Menlo Park, New Jersey. The authors wish to express their appreciation to Doctor Ralph Brancale, Medical Director of the New Jersey State Diagnostic Center, for permission to use the reported material and his interest and encouragement in this study.

Case 1: Mrs. A.

The couple was referred because of marital difficulties, and Mrs. A.'s complaints of her husband's infidelity. At the time of the examination, the husband was 51 years old, the wife 38 years old. Mr. A. was married once before, but he divorced his first wife after 14 years. The divorce was due to poor relations between the spouses. It was Mrs. A.'s first marriage, and she met Mr. A. when she was only 25 years old. The couple had been married for ten years at the time of the examination. Shortly after marriage, Mrs. A. became suspicious of her husband and on many occasions she left him, going to her mother's home and then coming back unexpectedly. This led to several short separations. A few months prior to the interview, her behavior became rather unreasonable. She claimed that another woman was coming to the house; she allegedly found nail polish on the garage door and lipstick on the toothpicks and on the towels. Sometimes on coming to the house she destroyed furniture, and on one occasion shot a BB gun in the house. Since she destroyed his furniture, Mr. A. was forced to put another lock on the door so that she could not get in with the old key.

In the office, during the interview, Mrs. A. was well-dressed, neatly groomed, friendly, and made a nice impression. She talked fluently, was able to give biographical data in good chronological order, and she was well oriented and in good contact with her surroundings. However, it became obvious that she acted under the influence of paranoid delusions. She was very circumstantial and she gave many details to illustrate her point. She produced towels and toothpicks with lipstick to prove "that another woman was coming to her house." She claimed it could not be her lipstick, since she stopped using it once she discovered that someone else was coming to the house. She claimed that she came back home unexpectedly to check on her husband, and when she came in he gave her a cold greeting, thus hurting her feelings. She also stopped having sexual relations with him, because she did not want to "share him with another woman." To substantiate her complaints, she stated that once she found a smudge of lipstick on the door of the bathroom, which she thought was done deliberately by the other woman in order to irritate her. On one occasion, she also found a "hair of another woman" on the visor of her husband's car. Later on, talking to the psychologist during psychological testing, she related that this hair "was a vaginal hair" and therefore she pulled a hair out of her pubic area and put it on the visor to "show the woman that she was still around."

In talking about the beginning of her marriage, she reported that girls greeted her husband, "Hello Bob" and asked him "if he will be there," thus implying that even then, ten years ago, he already was unfaithful to her. She also accused him of being oversexed, so much that her vagina became sore, and that he attempted to practice abnormal sex relations with her.

In this case, there is a great deal of pseudo-memories and paranoid delusions with erotic content. In spite of the fact that Mrs. A. was extremely disorganized, as far as her behavior and thinking are concerned, she may impress one, during a casual conversation, as an intelligent, interesting and charming woman. The towels and toothpicks with lipstick, which she produced as "evidence," should not mislead the wary. It was obvious the lipstick was from her own lips (in spite of her statement that she stopped using lipstick) since while in the office, her lips were thickly covered with it.

Case 2: Mrs. B.

Mrs. B., a 31-year-old mother of two children, married for approximately ten years, filed a complaint of inadequate support and requested inquiry into her marital status. The early part of the marital history was not remarkable, except that Mrs. B. had some difficulties with other women while following her husband to various Army camps during his military service. After his discharge from the service, the couple moved close to Mr. B.'s family. Mr. B. was, to some extent, dominated by his family and entered into a rather disadvantageous business venture with his brother. The real difficulties started seven years after marriage, shortly after the birth of the second child. Mrs. B. decided at first to sleep apart from her husband. This, however, was interrupted, off and on, by a week or so of a honeymoon relationship, but then again Mrs. B. slept apart in a different room and threatened to leave the house. She became more and more irritable and on many occasions was seen upset and crying. The husband's attempts to resume friendly relationships usually failed, and once when he asked if she wanted him to bring a cup of coffee, she answered, "I wouldn't be surprised if you put poison in this coffee."

Mrs. B. started complaining to neighbors about her husband's abusing and mistreating her. Her family physician was so impressed by her "woes" that he helped her contact a lawyer. When another physician, suspecting a mental disorder, sent the couple to a psychiatrist, the latter, after a short interview, declared that Mrs. B. "was of sound mind" and told the husband to treat his wife with more consideration. Meanwhile, Mrs. B. spread the news that she was in love with a man in the neighborhood, and she claimed that she went out with this man and his family to the seashore, since they were planning to be married. She talked about it without reserve to strangers and to her husband, who never saw his wife and the neighbor together, but nevertheless believed the story.

Mrs. B. was attractively attired and obviously tried to make an impression during the interview. Her speech was well-connected. She seemed to be lucid, cultured, intelligent and somewhat sophisticated. Since she was seen before her husband, her account gave the impression that one was dealing with a rather gifted woman who just was tired of her inadequate and insecure husband and of the domination of his immediate family. However, here and there, during the interview, she made sly remarks about her husband's intentions which put one on guard. In the beginning nothing, but her emphasis on her husband's rather peculiar preferences appeared (her husband later admitted that it was true), such as shaving her pubic hair, liking to bathe her, and occasionally insisting on cunnilingus and fellatio. Then, she reported that during one of their reconciliations he took her to a restaurant in New York where he acted "like a big shot" to impress her. She intimated that this invitation had some hidden meaning. She also reported that she found matches from a restaurant, again intimating that her husband, for some reason, spent his time away from home.

Mrs. B. was able to gain the sympathy of people she was in contact with; yet, her behavior was inconsistent. For instance, she related even to strangers the story of being in love with another man, at the same time filing a complaint of nonsupport by her husband. When his complaint was investigated by the judge, it was determined to be unfounded. The story of having gone out with another man was also unfounded and was probably what Kraepelin considered a "pseudomemory." Later on, further investigation showed that about a year earlier the husband had been brought home by a rescue squad after an automobile accident. Mrs. B. felt, at that time, that her husband was faking, and therefore she called the police station to find out whether there really had been an accident. In this case, no bizarre delusional material was elicited, but the patient expressed her delusional thinking by various intimations and remarks, seeing in simple events some kind of a hidden meaning.

Case 3: Mrs. C.

The couple was referred after Mrs. C. filed a complaint of nonsupport against her husband, charging that for the past several weeks he had virtually refused to support her. The marriage was the second for both Mr. and Mrs. C., and, at the time of the examination, Mrs. C. was 42 years old and her husband several years her senior. They had been married for approximately five years. Shortly after the marriage, Mrs. C. became extremely jealous of her husband. Even when he was at work, she spied on him. Mr. C., in relating his behavior, stated: "She was spying on me through the blinds. I thought at first she was interested in what I was doing." She also accused him of being friendly to his first wife and, on one occasion, she accused him of being a homosexual. She suspected that he was lying, going out with a girl in the neighborhood, and felt that he was not sufficiently potent sexually, "because he spent most of his sperm on other women." On one occasion, when he drove a truck with her sitting beside him, she suddenly said, "You don't love me," opened the door of the truck and attempted to jump out. She had frequent temper tantrums and, on one occasion, the husband slapped her "in order to get her out of hysterics."

About a year and a half before the examination, Mrs. C. complained that her husband did not support her adequately; however, according to the evidence, he supported her in keeping with his means. In the interview, the patient's brother disclosed that her immediate family was on her side, feeling that her husband abused her and did not support her properly.

The interview of Mrs. C. revealed a well-dressed, rather charming, pleasant, 42-year-old woman. She talked freely, her speech was coherent, she was well oriented, and could give biographical data in good chronological order. No psychotic material was elicited at the beginning of the interview when she related her biography, but little by little, ideas of a paranoid nature were brought to the surface. She made many intimations with a sly smile, made evasive statements, and reported definite pseudo-memories. For instance, she said five days after marriage, her husband hit her with a dish of food because she called him while he was out in the yard talking to a girl. The girl allegedly had a bad reputation in the neighborhood. At one time, when he took her to the family physician for an examination, he "made some signs to the physician," implying that she was insane. She could not invite her friends anymore, since she "was afraid" her "husband would make scenes." The friends who were coming to her home "had strange expressions" on their faces, and they acted as if "they heard some bad reports about her." She claimed that she found female clothes and towels from a hotel in his room. When asked why would he bring female clothes to his home, she answered: "Maybe he does it to upset me or to antagonize me." Then when asked why would he not openly admit to his activities with other women, she answered, "He's too shrewd for it. I know he doesn't love me and doesn't want me." She also accused her husband of stealing and actually attempting to kill her. On one occasion, she was standing on a street when a car passed very close to her. She felt that, in some way, this was connected with her husband's desire to get rid of her.

In this case, in spite of very definite delusional material elicited from the patient, neither her husband nor her immediate family suspected a psychosis. Her immediate family completely believed all her accusations. When this couple appeared before the judge, Mr. C. is quoted to have said, "I don't understand this whole thing myself. She never seems to be satisfied." In spite of quite severe personality disintegration, Mrs. C. could function socially, and could appear charming and interesting.

Case 4: Mrs. D.

Mrs. D. filed a complaint against her husband charging him with being cruel and abusive, using obscene language, making unusual sexual demands, and refusing to give her a cash allowance for necessities of life. At the time of the examination, both husband and wife were 28 years old, married for a period of five years, and the parents of four children. Shortly after their engagement, Mrs. D. wanted to return her ring to her fiancée, since she felt she was not worthy of him because of masturbation. Sexual relations were unsatisfactory from the very beginning. Six months after the marriage, Mrs. D. suggested divorce because she was "not good enough for her husband," again admitting masturbation before marriage, and a feeling that she would stand in her husband's way. A few days later, she attempted suicide by turning on the gas. Since then, she has made two additional attempts on her life by taking an overdose of sleeping medicine.

About two years before the examination, the D.'s became friendly with a young couple, the X.'s. At approximately that time, tension in the household was on the increase. Mrs. D. had frequent temper tantrums, became more argumentative than usual, and finally became suspicious of her husband's feelings for Mrs. X. Mrs. D. won the sympathy of her neighborhood, complaining to everybody about her husband's moral, physical, and sexual abuse and of his "affair" with Mrs. X. So skillful was Mrs. D. in winning the public's sympathy, that a neighborhood tavern owner advised his clients not to buy in Mr. D.'s store, since he "mistreated his wife" and "wanted to put her away." Mrs. D.'s immediate family was also aroused against Mr. D., hearing from Mrs. D. about her husband's alleged abuse and brutality. Mrs. D.'s sister, interviewed in the office, expressed a great deal of hostility toward her brother-in-law, and painted him as an exceedingly brutal and morally unworthy individual.

The examination of Mrs. D. revealed that she was a rather attractive and friendly young woman, well-oriented, giving a very convincing account of her "woes." In the beginning of the interview, while listening to her, it seemed that she was married to a brutal and emotionally disturbed individual. However, very soon statements with a delusional flavor were brought up. Her accusations were out of context and, at times, seemed to be improbable. For instance, she stated that at one time the X. couple slept in their house. Mrs. X. and Mr. D. woke up at night and allegedly went together to the children's room, implying that they had intercourse there. "Mrs. X.," she reported, "was dressed in a nightgown through which her pubic hair could be seen, and Mr. D. was in his pajamas." It is quite improbable that Mrs. X., who slept with her husband, in Mrs. D.'s home would leave the bed at night and meet with Mr. D. while her husband was sleeping, thus endangering the reputation of both. Furthermore, Mr. X. later sued Mrs. D. for slandering his wife.

There were also several other contradictory statements; for instance, she said that her husband's mother had told her about him and Mrs. X. being in love. Yet, shortly afterwards, talking about her mother-in-law, she accused her of calling her "insane" and "imagining things." She also reported events with an incorrect emphasis, implying that there was more in the event than it would seem. She reported in this context her husband's outcries, "Oh God! I'll kill you!" and "I don't love you anymore," when in reality this was nothing but a temper outburst aroused by her behavior. When later asked whether she really thought her husband actually wanted to kill her, she answered, "I don't know, but I do think he is trying to make me so upset I'll have a nervous breakdown and he will get rid of me and have the children." When asked why he made her nervous, she answered, "He cannot support me and the children, so I figured out if I stay calm and have my normal wits, he will not be able to remarry." She also intimated Mrs. X.'s child looks exactly like her husband.

In this case, in spite of a history of three suicide attempts, and rather strange behavior before and after marriage, the psychosis was not recognized. The neighborhood and the family were won over by Mrs. D., and finally Mr. D. became so disgruntled that he started staying away from home as much as he could. Thus, the patient's apparent lucidity and evidence of her husband's loss of interest misled many people. Yet, with a methodical psychiatric examination, it was possible to bring to the surface definite delusions (such as that Mrs. X.'s child looked like her husband), pseudo-memories (such as Mr. D.'s mother told her that he was in love with Mrs. X.), various inconsistencies, and rather poor judgment (such as "all this was done to make her nervous and get rid of her").

Case 5: Mrs. E.

The couple was referred because of marital discord. At the time of the examination, the husband was 40 years old, the wife 34 years old. When examined, the couple had been married 10 years. Difficulties started right after marriage. At first, Mrs. E. felt that it was abnormal to have sexual relations three times a week. She forced her husband to cut it to once a week. Later on, she felt that this was also abnormal and very frequently refused sexual relations, stating that she had her period. Several years ago, Mr. E. started a business of his own, but Mrs. E. did everything she could to ruin it. She started accusing him of having relations with a policeman's wife; she made scenes at home; at times, she did not let him in and he had to sleep at is place of business on the floor. She complained to the minister, to her lawyer, and to the policeman that her husband was a sex pervert, and later she accused most of the women in the neighborhood of being prostitutes. One morning when her husband went to the post office, and returned in 20 minutes, she accused him of having had intercourse with a girl who lived down the street. She also felt people were not neighborly, since she came from the South.

In the interview situation, Mrs. E. was pleasant, cooperative and talkative. Listening to her one could picture her husband as a stupid, bragging, and rather brutal individual in need of psychiatric care. Her account sounded plausible until she reported that her husband threatened to kill her. She accused him of situations for which she herself was responsible. Thus, she blamed her husband for sleeping in the store instead of coming home, when in reality she herself barred his entrance. She also accused him of being a sex pervert who forced her to perform fellatio. She claimed that he was going out with other women, and she made disparaging remarks about his claims of being a business man and, in general, did everything to show him in a poor light.

NOTES

1. 77 N.J. L.J. 299 (1954).
2. Revitch, E. (1954). The Problem of Conjugal paranoia, *Diseases of the Nervous System, 15*:271-277.
3. A delusion is a false belief without basis in reality, which cannot be changed by persuasion or even by positive proof to the contrary. For instance, a patient may believe that he is being persecuted, or is God, etc.
4. Kraepelin, E. (1921 ed.). *Manic-depressive insanity and paranoia.* Oxford: Livingstone, LRD.
5. An hallucination is a false sense perception without basis in reality. For example, hearing voices when no one is talking is an auditory hallucination.

6. The greater incidence of paranoia in the general population than reported, and the failure to diagnose the condition was stressed in Bonner, H. (1951). The problem of diagnosis in paranoic disorder, 107. *Am. J. of Psychiat., 677*:167-683.
7. Freud, S. (1948 ed). Psycho-analytic notes upon an autobiographical account of a case of paranoia (3) *Collected Papers of Sigmund Freud*.
8. Kraepelin, E. *op cit supra* note 4.
9. Meyer, A. (1951 ed.). Paranoia (2), *The Collected Papers of Adolph Meyer.*
10. Adler, A. (1946 ed.). *The practice and theory of individual psychology.*
11. In addition to the problem presented (litigation against the matrimonial relationship, created and maintained as a result of delusions of the patient), there is also the problem of the custody of the children, if separation or divorce is granted on other valid grounds. A paranoic mother or father can be a good parent, but as stated before, the derangement is psychotic, and hence, if there is a suspicion of the presence of such a condition, a complete psychiatric evaluation should be obtained before custody of a child is granted to the suspected parent.
12. Kraepelin, E. (1921). *op. cit supra* note 4, at pp. 216-217.
13. In New Jersey, the Juvenile and Domestic Relations Court, in dealing with matrimonial problems, has investigative powers and facilities, unavailable to the upper courts except in contested custody of children cases; (*Cf.* R. R. 6:3-8, 6:3-9, 6:2-11 (b), 6:5-5 and 4:98-8). These functions include marriage counseling, social investigations and psychiatric examinations, when marital discord problems occur, and the facts indicate to the judge the likelihood of a mental problem existing below the surface, a psychiatric examination at the State Di agnostic Center is recommended, usually for both parties. The result of such an examination, together with evaluations by the interviewing psychiatrist, are forwarded to the court for their use in disposing of the case. It was stated by Judge Libby E. Sachar of the Juvenile and Domestic Relations Court in Elizabeth, New Jersey, that an amazing and alarming number of marital partners involved in domestic discord have been found to be mentally ill. Many settlements are attributed to knowledge gained by psychiatric examinations in such cases.
14. 3 N. J. Misc. 576, 129 Atl. 122 (Ch. 1925).
15. 4o. N. J. Eq. 566, 5 Atl. 109 (Ct. Err. & App. 1885).
16. Mere insanity does not totally disqualify a person as a witness. The test for this generally is sufficient mental capacity to (1) observe a relevant matter, (2) correctly state these observations, and (3) appreciate the obligation to tell the truth under the sanctions locally imposed. As pertains to (1), a paranoic's views as to what is relevant may vary, but they must have sufficient mental capacity to observe such matters. As to (2), they may correctly state some of their observations, but more likely, as to observations regarding their marital affairs, they may exaggerate what they saw, or state facts which they in reality never saw, but firmly believe they did see (i.e., pseudo-memories). In all events, the interpretations they place on the alleged observations, which, in turn, they re-lated as facts, will directly result from the delusions from which they suffer. If the cross-examiner can make his witness divulge what these observations mean to

him (i.e., his interpretations of the alleged facts), there is a good chance that, in most cases, the reply will be of such a delusional nature and so illogical that the paranoid condition will have been exposed.

17. *Cf.* R. R. 4:93-2, 4:25-1, 4:25-2 as to actions in the Superior Court, and R. R. 6:3-8 as to those in the Juvenile and Domestic Relations Court.
18. Frank, J. (1953). Judicial fact finding and psychology, 14 *Ohio ST. L. J.*, 183.
19. N. J. STAT. 2A:34-2 and 2A:34-3.

Chapter 13

DIAGNOSIS AND DISPOSITION OF THE PARANOID MARITAL PARTNER

A latent psychosis, with paranoid symptomatology in one of the spouses, was a frequent cause of conjugal discord in couples referred for psychiatric evaluation to the New Jersey State Diagnostic Center by the domestic relations courts. This syndrome was found in 39 out of 93 (41%) of the couples that I evaluated at the Diagnostic Center. Only isolated cases were encountered in private practice. The difference is probably due to the fact that marital difficulties, connected with other causes, are not generally referred to psychiatrists, but may be seen by marriage counselors. The paranoid partners rarely submit, of their own free will, to psychiatric examination. There is a whole spectrum of paranoid conditions, with lesser or greater personality disorganization, ranging from true paranoia[1] to the paranoid form of schizophrenia.

Paranoid states with good personality organization involving only, or mostly, the marital partner in their delusional system were described as conjugal paranoia[2,3] and as the Othello syndrome.[4] The basic symptomatology consists of accusations of infidelity, destructive, hostile, and domineering attitudes toward the spouse, coupled with inner insecurity and basic dependency on the marital partner. The diagnostic difficulties are due to excellent preservation of the patient's personality and the ability of being convincing to others. By means of rationalization and projection, reality is distorted to such an extent that not the patient, but the marital partner, may be suspected of being abnormal. Very often the patient's accusations are based on some truth. For instance,

Source: Revitch, E. (1960). Diagnosis and disposition of the paranoid marital partner. *Diseases of the Nervous System, 21*:117-118.

the wife may accuse the husband of hitting her. Indeed, he may have hit her, but it was provoked by her unreasonable accusations and disruptive behavior. On occasions, the patients fabricate "evidence." Thus, one male patient inflicted bruises on his chest and took colored slides as proof that his wife had hit him. Once I was consulted by a husband who asked that I commit his wife to a state hospital. She broke the radio, tore his shirt, and lay motionless in bed. In talking to the neighbors and the wife, I found out about his pathological jealousy, constant accusations of infidelity and his bizarre behavior. Thus, he would not allow her to go to the bathroom at night, since he believed that men would watch her through the bathroom window. Her behavior was considered by him to be an outburst of temper produced by his accusations.

I have examined several cases in which the sick spouse was given a clean bill of health, while the partner was accused by the physician of being brutal, unfaithful, or even suffering from a paranoid state. These patients frequently convince the families, neighbors, and even the police of the veracity of their distortions, so that the marital partner may suffer. Thus, the husband of one of the patients was not allowed by the police to follow his wife to the state hospital, since it was felt the woman had been unjustly "put away." In many cases, the paranoid spouse was known to be gentle and considerate during courtship. However, at the beginning of marital life, frequently during the honeymoon, there are instances of disparaging remarks, humiliating attitudes, accusations of infidelity, as well as disinterest and disregard for the partner's needs and feelings. Accusations of infidelity may occur in the beginning only in spots, and the spouse may even later retract these accusations as a joke or as statements made in anger. Later the accusations become a firm belief and thus acquire the characteristics of delusions.

In addition to accusations of infidelity, there may be accusations of homosexuality or incest, or sexual perversions and insanity. Yet, it is the accusing partner himself who shows symptoms of delayed or conflicted psychosexual maturation. Thus, he or she may show interest in pornography, fellatio, cunnilingus, masturbation, rectal intercourse, and so forth, while accusing others of being sexually abnormal. The refusal of the partner to submit to the patient's sexual whims will sometimes lead to outbursts of rage with choking, spitting, and physical abuse, particularly in cases where the male spouse is the paranoiac. There may also be checking of the spouse's whereabouts and of the underclothing, allegedly to find a trace of lipstick or of semen. Alcoholism is frequently, but not always, associated with this condition.

In order to avoid grave diagnostic errors, it is not sufficient to see one spouse. Both spouses should always be examined separately and then in a joint interview. In a joint interview both are confronted, and a laboratory condition of the marital relationship is created. This permits the psychiatrist to clarify the contradictory and misleading statements, as well as the affective relationship of both spouses. In one instance, the paranoid wife complained that her husband did not come home and slept in his place of business, thus rejecting her. The joint interview, however, revealed that she did not let him get into the house, so that he found it necessary to sleep in his store.

Accusations of infidelity in cases of conjugal paranoia should be differentiated from pathological jealousy of weak, insecure, and possessive persons. In the latter cases, the spouse is appreciated but, due to the patient's insecurity, he or she has to be constantly reassured of being loved. The possessiveness and the love needs of these patients are so intense that they constantly feel dissatisfied and suspicious. They constantly torture themselves and their partners, yet they genuinely desire harmony and faithfulness. In conjugal paranoia, on the contrary, accusations of infidelity seem to serve the purpose of proving the spouse to be amoral or inferior. In some cases, the partner is induced by the patient to commit adultery.

As long as the paranoid patients function well enough to support the family, I usually do not recommend commitment. However, in cases of threats to the life of the spouse, or in cases of extreme disorganization of the family, commitment is necessary. Unfortunately, the hospital personnel do not always recognize the delusional nature of the patient's thinking and commitment often will be followed by rapid discharge, or what is worse, the patient may not be declared psychotic and will be thrown back to the family while harboring undisclosed homicidal preoccupations. Attempts at reconciliation are futile and aggravate the problem. Separation of spouses usually improves the well-being of the family. Under no circumstances should the healthy spouse be advised to give in to the whims of the paranoid partner. Firm attitudes and personal independence are more likely to succeed in normalizing the situation. Thus, in one case where the wife was ready to give up a job she liked, hoping to please the husband and allay his suspicions, a good effect was produced by helping her to become independent.

I have never been able to establish a therapeutic relationship with the paranoid spouse. The weak and dependent persons with pathological jealousy, on the contrary, may seek therapy and particularly reassurance. They are willing and able to be helped and to gain insight. There is, however, a danger of misdiagnosing the sufferers with pathological jealousy as cases of conjugal paranoia. This is of more than academic interest since treatment and prognosis is different in both cases. While in conjugal paranoia the prognosis is poor, and separation should be recommended, in most cases, in pathological jealousy of insecure individuals, psychotherapy may be successful. The danger of misdiagnosing the healthy spouse as paranoic or mentally ill can be avoided only by a thorough and unhurried interview of both spouses individually and in a joint session. The Rorschach and other projective techniques frequently do not reveal the psychotic process and thus cannot be relied upon for a definitive diagnosis.

REFERENCES

1. Kraepelin, E. (1921). *Manic-depressive insanity and paranoia.* Edinburg: E. andS. Livingstone.
2. Revitch, E. (1954). The problem of conjugal paranoia. *Dis. of Nerv. Syst., 15*:271.
3. Revitch, E., & Hayden, J. W. (1955). Paranoid marital partner: Counselor's client, psychiatrist's problem. *Rutgers Law Review, 9*:512.
4. Todd, J., and Dewhurst, K. (1955). The Othello Syndrome. *J. of Nerv. and Ment. Dis., 122*:367.

Section III

PSYCHIATRIC ASPECTS OF EPILEPSY AND EPILEPTOID VIOLENCE

INTRODUCTION

"Epilepsy frequently involves the borderland area [of neurology and psychiatry] since more often than any other neurological condition, it [epilepsy] has intrinsic connections with psychiatric problems in the differential diagnosis, symptomatology and social adjustment" (Revitch, 1982, p. 11). Although Doctor Revitch practiced primarily as a psychiatrist, he developed an intense interest in neurology while still in medical school. Once he finished his psychiatric residency, he took additional training in neurology, with a focus on epilepsy. He was truly an epileptologist, specializing particularly in what has been referred to as the "borderland" area where neurology and psychiatry intersect. Even when two specialists communicate with each other about the same patient, Doctor Revitch believed that two specialists do not replace one clinician grounded in both specialties, notwithstanding the impossibility of equal competence in both disciplines.

In the first chapter in Section III, Doctor Revitch outlines psychiatric problems found in the diagnosis and treatment of epilepsy. He describes a number of illustrative cases and highlights topics such as epileptic personality, epileptic deterioration, and the various social-adjustment problems epileptics encounter.

In Chapter 15, various epileptic manifestations that resemble psychiatric disorders are covered. Too often, true epileptic seizures are misdiagnosed as being purely psychiatric. Doctor Revitch provides a number of cases and he notes especially the limitations of the EEG as a diagnostic tool. "Electroencephalography is not as well standardized as electrocardiography and therefore one encounters many so-called borderline records" (Revitch, 1956, p. 1058). Instead of heavy reliance solely on the EEG, he stresses the benefits of a careful and unhurried history. In Chapter 16, Doctor Revitch further discusses diagnostic problems in epilepsy. He reviews different methods of diagnosis, and problems involving brain tumors, febrile seizures, as well as petit mal and minor seizures. Abdominal symptoms in epilepsy–often missed not only by neurologists and psychiatrists, but sometimes by internists as well–are also reviewed.

In Chapter 17, Doctor Revitch discusses psychomotor paroxysms of nonepileptic origin. This 1958 paper provides an interesting presentation of hysterical dissociation, rage reactions, as well as autonomic and psychic emotional discharges. The chapter also includes a fascinating discussion of Doctor Revitch's paper by six leading authorities in the field. In Chapter 18, Doctor Revitch further describes paroxysmal manifestations of a nonepileptic origin--which he referred to as catathymic attacks. He describes catathymic outbursts, and the differential diagnosis, etiology, and the mechanism of such emotional outbursts. Catathymic explosions are considered to be strong and often violent emotional releases, a concept that he further developed during the following 30 years.

Psychomotor paroxysms of nonepileptic, as well as epileptic, origin are discussed in Chapter 19. The differential diagnosis between epilepsy and nonepileptic explosive outbursts highlights the problem of the complete separation between psychiatry and neurology. Doctor Revitch supports a neuropsychiatric approach rather than separate psychiatric or purely neurological perspectives, especially in these difficult and often ambiguous cases. Accordingly, he advises physicians, who at that time had to report cases of epilepsy to boards of health, not to list patients as epileptic just because of the paroxysmal nature of their condition, which may be purely emotionally based.

In the final chapter of this section, Doctor Revitch discusses the social aspects of epilepsy. This paper, one of Doctor Revitch's earliest, published in 1951, stresses the need to give epileptic patients guidance with respect to their understanding of the illness, the need to foster a feeling of self-esteem in epileptic patients, and the need to change public attitudes towards epilepsy. He argues that not only physicians but social workers and others should stress–through the press, radio, and other media–the truth about various aspects of epilepsy and should also dispel myths about the disorder.

REFERENCES

Revitch, E. (1956). Diagnostic problems in epilepsy. *Medical Times: The Journal of General Practice, 84*:1056-1065.

Revitch, E. (1982). Psychiatric problems in epilepsy. *Family Practice Journal of JFK Medical Center, Spring*:11-14.

Chapter 14

PSYCHIATRIC PROBLEMS IN EPILEPSY

The complete separation of psychiatry and neurology has created a borderline area which is largely neglected by both specialties. Mark[1] deplores lack of communication between the neurologist and the psychiatrist treating the same patient. It has been my contention for a long time that this type of collaboration between the two specialties cannot replace the overall neuropsychiatric perspective of one clinician grounded in both disciplines. It must be recognized, however, that in view of the rapid progress of medical knowledge and technology, equal competence in both disciplines is an impossibility. Therefore, certain specific technical problems in the borderland area should be surrendered to the specialist with greater knowledge and experience. Epilepsy frequently involves the borderland area since more often than any other neurological condition, it has intrinsic connections with psychiatric problems in the differential diagnosis, symptomatology, and social adjustment.

DIAGNOSTIC PROBLEMS

It is easy to diagnose the well-known classical grand mal seizures. However, there are complex seizures, dominated by psychological and behavioral manifestations, which may be of epileptic or nonepileptic origin. Epilepsy is a clinical correlate of an excessive neuronal discharge in the brain as conceived of by J. Hughlings Jackson over a century ago. The varieties of the nonepileptic seizures or pseudoseizures[1-6] can be conceived as falling on a spectrum of purely

---

Source: Revitch, E. (1982). Psychiatric problems in epilepsy. *Family Practice Journal of JFK Medical Center. Spring*:11-14.

physiological causes (such as hypoglycemia) through a mixture of psychological and physiological causes such as fainting spells and cataplectic attacks in narcolepsy), and finally, purely psychological causes such as hysterical seizures.

The clinical EEG, introduced by Hans Berger in the early 1930s, and later electrocorticography and the use of depth electrodes in neurosurgery or epilepsy and in experimental conditions,[7] amply confirmed the Jacksonian concept. The EEG is a necessary adjunct to the diagnostic armamentarium, but unfortunately the abnormal discharge is not always detected in the usual clinical practice with the use of scalp electrodes. Furthermore, epileptiform discharges may be found in the EEGs of nonepileptics. This is particularly confusing, in cases of abnormal records, in the nonepileptic seizures. A combination of epileptic and nonepileptic seizures in the same patient has been amply documented, and this again complicates and confuses the diagnostic problem.

The greatest problem in diagnosis, however, is complex seizures with the dominance of psychological and behavioral manifestations. Paroxysmality is the hallmark of all the seizures, but loss of complete awareness of the surroundings may be absent in the complex epileptic seizures. To the contrary, it may be present or, at least, claimed in the nonepileptic seizures.

Williams[8] explains the difficulty in differentiating behavioral and psychic phenomena of complex epileptic seizures from purely psychiatric conditions in the following words: "The higher the level of cerebral function involved in the epileptic disturbance, the more likely it is to have continuity with and be patterned by pre-ictal events, a situation not encountered in simple epilepsies."

Lennox[9] cites the case of a young man who had brutally murdered his favorite aunt and claimed amnesia for the event. This man had a history of two convulsions in childhood and a history of brutal assaults on playmates and siblings. Soft neurological signs, including reflex changes on the right side, with spiking in the left temporal lobe in the EEG record, convinced one of the experts that the murder had been committed during a psychomotor seizure. Lennox, however, was more cautious and he left the diagnosis unresolved, since the subject had no seizures and he was well behaved during the seven years of follow-up in prison.

The following five cases previously reported[3,10] will illustrate the complexity of the problem.

Case 1

Following World War II, I treated a 30-year-old patient in a Veteran's Administration hospital for unstable behavior with attacks of flushing of the face, falling down, thrashing of arms and legs, and resisting those who attempted to restrain him. He carried various psychiatric diagnoses ranging from hysteria to psychopathic personality and schizophrenia.

Only after several interviews with the patient was I able to discover that the attacks were preceded by a feeling of surge in epigastrium followed by a visual aura. This type of aura is typical in temporal lobe seizures. Only after several normal EEGs had been recorded, was left temporal spiking elicited in light sleep. Eight years later, I saw him again at the New Jersey State Diagnostic Center through court referral because of incestuous conduct with his daughter. He then claimed that following the termination of a stormy marriage his attacks stopped in spite of failure to continue on anticonvulsive medication.

Case 2

A veteran in his mid-thirties was seen and followed in the same facility as the previous case, and then 10 years later I saw him as a private patient for one year. After his ship had been torpedoed, he developed inner tension and irritability. While on leave from a naval hospital, he had his first attack of destructive violence which necessitated forceful restraint.

Only after considerable follow-up was it clarified that the attacks of violence with hazy memory for the event were preceded by progressively mounting tension, anger, headaches, depression, crying spells, and fleeting paranoid misinterpretations of surrounding incidents. This usually lasted several days. Following the violent and destructive attack which lasted perhaps half an hour, he felt guilty, depressed, and suicidal for several days. His marriage was stormy and pathological. Thus, he forced his wife to sexually entice men and to have sexual relations with women. His attacks stopped following the dissolution of his marriage. Originally his EEG revealed left temporal spiking, but I could not elicit this 10 years later.

Case 3

A 28-year-old veteran developed attacks involving feelings of impending doom, faintness, profuse perspiration, general haziness of consciousness, goose pimples, cold and clammy extremities, rapid heartbeats, and bloating and shrinking feelings in the epigastrium. This was preceded by flushing of the face. A day or two before the attack he felt restless, aggressive, and depressed. Independent of the attacks, he experienced a compulsion to stab people with a knife. This lasted for several days and was accompanied by an effort to resist the urge. This condition was preceded by his brother's accidental death. A five per second flat top wave pattern with six per second positive spikes in both temporal lobes was elicited. Seizures stopped with anticonvulsive medication. He had been treated previously as a purely psychiatric case carrying various psychiatric diagnoses.

Case 4

A 17-year-old boy was referred to the New Jersey State Diagnostic Center for evaluation of episodes of blind destructive range and with what seemed like a loss of awareness of the environment. The attacks were triggered by trivial events. The EEG and neurological studies were entirely within normal limits. In the psychiatric interviews, he disclosed severe feelings of inferiority and dizziness, nausea, tension, and hyperventilation preceding the attacks.

Case 5

A 19-year-old inmate of a female reformatory was examined and followed for outbursts of seemingly unprovoked and uncontrollable rage, including falling down to the ground and what looked like loss of consciousness. The diffuse burst-like activity in the EEG suggested epilepsy, and she had been actually treated with anticonvulsives without success.

In light hypnosis and under I.V. sodium amytal, she revealed distrust of people and, at the most trivial provocation, she developed attacks of hyperventilation which were followed by loss of consciousness and falling down. She felt that she could stop the attacks if she let herself cry. The attacks improved when she received the news of a favorable parole action.

I saw her again 10 years later in my office. At that time her life was organized and she no longer had the attacks. A question arises as to whether these attacks were correlates of an excessive neuronal discharge (i.e., epileptic), or whether they were emotionally released phenomena.

EMOTIONAL FACTORS AND PSEUDO-SEIZURES

Gibbs and Gibbs[11] described attacks of rage, headaches and autonomic discharges accompanied by 6 and 14 per second spikes in the temporal lobes under the name of thalamic and hypothalamic epilepsy. Many epileptologists, however, believe that these attacks are not epileptic but emotional release phenomena, and that the normal EEG findings just point to a physiological focus of minor resistance which weakens the coping ability of the subject.

It seems to me that this reasoning should apply to Cases 2 and 5. Case 4 had a normal EEG. The seizures in Cases 1 and 3 were emotionally triggered, but I believe that they were of epileptic origin (temporal aura in Case 1 and a positive response to Dilantin in Case 3).

Emotional stimuli may lower the convulsive threshold and thus precipitate a seizure.[12] Other precipitating causes may be flashing lights in certain types of light-sensitive, usually petit mal, attacks. In fact, some children voluntarily precipitate such seizures by waving their hands in front of the eyes while looking at a light, which produces a flickering effect. In other cases, a seizure can be precipitated by stimulation of a part of the body which corresponds to the cortical area with a discharging epileptogenic focus. Reading, music, recollection, and revisualization of sights or events may cause temporal lobe seizures in some cases.[7] In some cases, a seizure may be aborted through mental concentration and various sensory stimuli. This was already mentioned by Gowers[13] and J. Hughlings Jackson at the turn of the century. There may be relatively silent epileptogenic foci in the temporal lobe, or in the limbic structures, which occasionally will fire under strong stimuli. This is the reason why in some cases of pseudo-seizures an occasional epileptic seizure may occur.

The hysterical seizures are, however, a purely psychiatric event and, as such, in cases of combined seizures, they imitate their epileptic attacks. The attacks of hysterical seizures with typical thrashing around, dramatic postures and arching of the back, as described by Charcot, are rare at present.

In the French literature pseudo-seizures, not considered to be hysterical but emotional release phenomena, are described under the name of "crises neuropathiques"[14] and "crises catathymiques."[15] Monroe's[16] episodic behavioral disorders cut across these cases except that they are connected with abnormal EEG records with administration of alpha-chloralose. Episodes of depersonalization, of macropsia and micropsia, of dysperception of changes of body scheme, and of an illusion of acceleration of body functions and of environmental events, may pose the differential diagnosis with temporal lobe seizures. These attacks occur mostly in states of isolation and inattention in a quiet environment.[2] A 13-year-old boy with illusions of acceleration could stop the episodes just by turning on the radio.

Gowers[13] placed what he called vaso-vagal attacks in the borderland of epilepsy. These attacks were manifested by tachycardia, feelings of suffocation, nausea, hot and cold flashes, pallor, sweating, shivering, and a feeling of agonizing fear. Gowers' vaso-vagal attacks were mostly somatic manifestations of anxiety which may sometimes look like ictal events.

At times, however, similar attacks may be of epileptic origin. Thus, Penfield[17] described under the name of diencephalic epilepsy attacks of sweating, gooseflesh, hypertension, pallor, flushing and fever. One of my patients whom I had previously treated for depression, developed attacks of tension, feelings of unreality and remoteness, tearing, and increases in blood pressure. These attacks lasted a few minutes and usually occurred during menses. Pheochromacytoma was at first suspected by her internist. Her EEGs in states of alertness and in sleep, with pharyngeal electrode placements, were negative. She improved with administration of Tegretol. I believe that this is a case of diencephalic epilepsy.

In temporal lobe or psychomotor epilepsy, recently renamed partial seizures with complex symptomatology, psychic aura of depression, anxiety, visual, auditory and olfactory aura are well-known. Weil,[18] however, described episodes of depression and anxiety with confusion in patients with temporal lobe lesions. In temporal lobe and in petit mal status epileptics, long-standing periods of confusion, psychotic behavior and fugues, suggestive of a purely psychiatric condition, have been described.[19] Interictal behavior disturbances in temporal lobe epileptics,[20] and schizophrenic-like psychosis late in the illness,[21] have been amply documented.

Epileptic Personality

Only few investigators currently believe that epileptics are endowed with specific personality traits. This view, however, was current at the turn of the century, when the concept of epileptic personality was popular. This was probably due to the fact that the experience of psychiatrists who described the syndrome was confined mainly to institutional cases.

Indeed, one can still find, in such cases, the characteristics described in epileptic personality: moodiness, temper tantrums, sensitivity, religiosity, perseveration and inability to shift affect (stickiness of affect). Sudden religious conversions in temporal lobe epileptics have been described in the literature.[22]

Epileptic Deterioration

Only a minority of epileptics deteriorate intellectually. In fact, history abounds with names of great men and creative geniuses who suffered from epilepsy. These include Julius Caesar, Flaubert, Dostoyevsky, and Van Gogh, just to cite a few. The earlier the onset of seizures, and the greater their frequency, the more likely there will be some deterioration. For this reason, there is some concern with small children who develop febrile seizures. Large amounts of medication may cause reversible suppression of cognitive faculties. Many seemingly deteriorated epileptics are actually brain damaged, or have an organic brain condition which causes both the seizures and the intellectual deterioration. This may be associated with unstable, impulsive and explosive behavior which may be alleviated by adding Mellaril to the anticonvulsive medication.

Social Adjustment

Prejudice against epileptics is widespread.[23] Caveness et al.[24] found that in 1949, 53 percent of their sample of the general population believed that epileptics were employable, but in 1969, 76 percent believed that epileptics should be employed. This is an indication of improved public attitudes. Perr[25] stated that attitudes toward epileptics reflect a lack of knowledge as well as attitudes "fixed into our cultural pattern by a legal system which has singled out epilepsy." Only within the past two decades has New Jersey abolished the antiquated statutes forbidding the marriage of epileptics and forcing physicians to report them to the local boards of health.

At present, epileptics have to be reported to the motor vehicle department, and they are allowed to drive after two years of freedom from seizures. The inability to drive, for those with seizures, limits their job opportunities. A seizure in public, or on a date, will cause embarrassment and will limit socialization. Imagine an adolescent counting the months and the days when he will be allowed to drive suddenly getting a seizure! Disbelief, anger, and refusal to cooperate–and to take medication–is common in these cases.

There is also an erroneous belief that epileptics are aggressive and that they are prone to crime and violence. According to some reports, there are more epileptics in prison than in the general population. This, however, is due to the fact that the bulk of prisoners come from lower socioeconomic strata of the population, with a history of neglect, deprivation, injuries and poor prenatal and postnatal care. Most of the crimes committed by epileptics are not due to epilepsy. Violence in ictal and post-ictal confusion is rare. Therefore, Crichton[26] was criticized for his book *The Terminal Man*, which would suggest violence to be the main characteristic of temporal lobe epilepsy.

COMMENT

This paper was conceived as an introduction into the psychiatric problems of epilepsy as well as to alert the reader to the borderland areas of psychiatry, and to the fact that neither psychiatry nor any other specialty should or can be detached from the rest of medicine. It is obvious that in addition to the intricate diagnostic problems and to the administration of anticonvulsives, there is also a problem of supportive guidance, follow-up and empathic understanding of the patient's overall problems of adjustment and of the worries and concern of his or her parents in the case of a child. A family physician with his or her global approach to medicine should be able to deal with the totality of the case, surrendering special problems to the proper consultants.

REFERENCES

1. Mark, V. (1979). The interface between psychiatry and neurology. *Psychiatric Opinion, 16*:39.
2. Revitch, E. (1966). Episodes of inattention and perceptual alteration. *Diseases of the Nervous System, 27*:789-794.
3. Revitch, E. (1964). Paroxysmal manifestations of non-epileptic origin: catathymic attacks. *Diseases of the Nervous System, 25*:662-669.
4. Revitch, E. (1970). Epileptic and non-epileptic paroxysms. *The Journal of the Medical Society of New Jersey, 67*:635-638.
5. Ferris, G. S. (1959). The recognition of non-epileptic seizures. *Southern Medical Journal, 52*:1557-1567.
6. Massey E. W., & Riley T. L. (1980). Pseudo-seizures: recognition and treatment. *Psychosomatics, 21*:1987-997.
7. Penfield W, & Jasper H. (1954). *Epilepsy and the functional anatomy of the human brain.* Boston; Little, Brown Co.
8. Williams, D. (1956). The structure of emotions reflected in epileptic experience. *Brain, 79*:29-67.
9. Lennox, W. G. (1960). *Epilepsy and related disorders*, Vol. II. Boson; Little, Brown and Co.
10. Revitch, E. (1954). Epileptic manifestations resembling psychiatric disorders. *Journal of the Medical Society of New Jersey, 51*:3-10.
11. Gibbs, E., & Gibbs, F. (1951). Electroencephalographic evidence of thalamic and hypothalamic epilepsy. *Neurology, 1*:136-144.
12. Lennox, W. G. (1944). Seizure states in personality and behavior disorders, Chap. 31. In: Hunt, J. *Personality and behavior disorders.* New York: Ronald Press.
13. Gowers, W. R. (1906). Clinical lectures on the borderland of epilepsy. *British Medical Journal*, 1617-1622.
14. Baruk, H. (1959). *Traite de Psychiatre, vol II.* Paris: Masson.
15. Gayral, L., Millet, G., Moron, P., & Turnin, J. (1956). Crises et paroxysms catathymiques. *Annales Medico-Psychologiques, 114*:25-50.
16. Monroe, R. R. (1974). Episodic behavioral disorders: An unclassified syndrome. In: Arieti S: *American Handbook of Psychiatry Vol II.* New York: Basic Books.
17. Penfield, W. (1929). Diencephalic autonomic epilepsy. *Archives of Neurology and Psychiatry, 22*:358-373.
18. Weil, A. (1956). Ictal depression and anxiety in temporal lobe disorders. *American Journal of Psychiatry, 113*:149-157.
19. Weiser, H. G. (1980). Temporal lobe of psychomotor status epilepticus: case report. *Electroencephalography and Clinical Neurophysiology, 18*: 558-572.
20. Gibbs, F. A. (1951). Ictal and non-ictal psychiatric disorders in temporal-lobe epilepsy. *Journal of Nervous and Mental Diseases, 113*:522-528.
21. Slater, E., & Beard, A. W. (1963). The schizophrenic-like psychoses in epilepsy: psychiatric aspects. *British Journal of Psychiatry, 109*:95-112.

22. Dewhurst, K., & Beard, A. W. (1970). Sudden religious conversions in temporal lobe epileptics. *British Journal of Psychiatry, 117*:497-507.
23. Bagley, C. (1972). Social prejudice and the adjustment of people with epilepsy. *Epilepsy, 13*:33-45.
24. Caveness, W., Merritt, H., & Gallup, G. (1969). *A Survey of Public Attitudes Toward Epilepsy in 1969.* Bethesda, MD: U.S. Department of Health, Education and Welfare: National Institutes of Health.
25. Perr, I. N. (1959). Epilepsy and the law. *Journal of Nervous and Mental Diseases, 28*:262-275.
26. Crichton, M. (1972). *The Terminal Man.* New York: Knopf.

Chapter 15

EPILEPTIC MANIFESTATIONS RESEMBLING PSYCHIATRIC DISORDERS

About 80 years, ago the English neurologist J. Hughlings Jackson defined epilepsy as a manifestation of excessive neuronal discharge. This concept was confirmed by the introduction of clinical electroencephalography by Hans Berger in the early 1930s. Electroencephalography has, however, limitations as a diagnostic tool. This is because normal interseizure electroencephalograms may be found in epileptics,[1,2] and abnormal epileptic-like patterns have been described by various investigators in nonepileptic prison inmates,[3,4] in children with behavior disorders,[5] in persons who committed motiveless murder,[6] and in relatives of epileptics. Furthermore, the tracing is not always specific for a particular type of epilepsy except, perhaps, the three per second wave spike complex described by Lennox[7] in the petit mal triad. The relative lack of specificity of the tracings, the existence of "borderline records," and the strong psychogenic orientation in modern psychiatry are frequently responsible for failure to recognize the less known, at times bizarre, paroxysmal phenomena whose epileptic nature is overlooked, and a purely psychiatric diagnosis is frequently given. These phenomena are as follows: (1) aborted grand mal or psychomotor seizures, (2) episodes of behavioral disorganization with or without dissolution of consciousness, (3) phenomena related to the activity of the automatic nervous system with or without psychic manifestations, and (4) akinetic seizures.

Source: Revitch, E. (1954). Epileptic manifestations resembling psychiatric disorders. *Journal of the Medical Society of New Jersey, 51*:3-10.

ABORTED GRAND MAL AND PSYCHOMOTOR SEIZURES

Two misdiagnoses are frequent. First, patients with grand mal seizures, particularly under treatment, develop very short attacks without frothing at the mouth, falling down and other textbook symptoms. The whole seizure may be over while the patient is seated; usually, after a short period of hazy consciousness, he is ready to resume his activities. Quite often, these seizures are described by nurses and doctors as "petit mal." Yet, the differential diagnosis is more than academic interest since the drugs of the hydantoin group (Dilantin, Mesantoin) are specific for grand mal seizures but usually are contraindicated in petit mal attacks. The reverse is true for the drugs of the oxasolidine-dione group (Tridione, Paradione). The diagnosis should be made on the presence or absence of a three per second wave spike complex in the electroencephalograms.

Second, the aura may constitute the whole seizure. Aura, which means breeze in Greek, was first described by Galen in one of his patients as tingling sensations in the extremities of one side preceding a grand mal seizure. Since Galen, all the "warning signs" of a seizure have been known as aura. However, if the seizure is viewed physiologically as a progressive invasion of the brain by the "excessive neuronal discharge," the aura will no longer be a "warning sign" of the seizure, but the beginning of the seizure itself. It will be a clinical translation of the "excessive neuronal discharge" at the discharging focus. It is obvious that if, for various reasons, the discharge stops at the focus and fails to spread over the rest of the brain, the patient will experience only the aura without the rest of the seizure. This particular point was extensively reviewed by Antoni[8] to whose paper the interested reader is referred. The auras referrable to the temporal lobe focus present a varied picture and are as follows: (1) olfactory hallucinations, (2) visual disturbances such as macropsia, micropsia, split in the visual field and formed visual hallucinations, (3) feelings of depersonalization, and (4) feelings of change of size and weight of various parts of the body.

Case 1

L. L., age 40 years, has had nocturnal seizures for several years. During the day, he experienced various sensations which were diagnosed as conversion hysteria and later schizophrenia. The fact that he had nocturnal seizures was not taken seriously since several electroencephalograms were perfectly normal. The patient, however, was extremely preoccupied by his sensations and, in despair, kept an accurate diary for a period of three years, with the hope that this would shed light on his condition. The description at times was so characteristic, that several excerpts of his diary will be transcribed here.

"Had that odd feeling again. Starts in the pit of the stomach and a sickening surge upward . . . On my travels, began feeling funny. Children coming from school seemed rather hazy and not more than 50 feet away. . . . While walking over to Mary's, I had a rather uncomfortable few minutes. Started in the same way, but with this difference. Fifth Street is lined with large trees about every 30-40 feet. As I approached a tree, it would vanish, then when I passed it, the next tree would vanish. I tried turning my head from side to side, but it did no good. Oh yes! Chills and goose flesh on my arms, with hair on my arms erect. When I reached Mary's, I found the same thing. Portions of her body looked invisible. But this finally wore off, leaving me uncomfortable."

EPISODES OF DISORGANIZED BEHAVIOR

Episodes of disorganized behavior with dissolution of consciousness are known, at the present time, under the name psychomotor epilepsy. Since a discharging focus in the temporal lobe is usually responsible for psychomotor attacks, auras referable to the discharge of this area are frequent. Gibbs et al.[9] described, in 1948, a more or less specific electroencephalographic pattern consisting of negative spikes in the anterior temporal region. The spike is either unilateral or bilateral, and there is phase reversal in other leads if the ear lobe is used as a reference point. This pattern is more frequent when the record is taken in light sleep and may be missed in deep sleep or when the patient is awake. The attacks may be of a rather simple pattern such as repetitive aimless movements, or may consist of furor, assaultiveness, or fugues. All of these activities, however, are amnesic and awareness during the attack is not preserved. Since many cases of psychomotor epilepsy also show interictal schizophrenic-like or psychopathic-like manifestations, and since the routine electroencephalograms may be either normal or without the specific pattern more commonly seen in sleep, diagnostic failures are more frequent than one may suspect.

Case 2

R. S., a 30-year-old male, gave a history of irresponsible, shiftless and aggressive behavior since childhood. For several years, he had attacks of falling down, rolling on the floor with aimless flailing of the extremities, and fighting those who approached him. Each seizure starts with an ill-defined sensation in the epigastrium and with a feeling of surge from his feet to his head. Then, shortly before the dissolution of consciousness, he experiences a vision of a candle surrounded by a halo. The halo gets smaller and then he no longer has any recollection of what follows. He has a feeling that by grabbing an object with his hands, he is able to fight off an attack, but he fails to remember whether he had ever been successful in preventing one. The patient has had several admissions to mental hospitals, and each time he was given diagnoses such as schizophrenia, psychopathic personality or reactive depression. His attacks were considered by many observers as either hysterical manifestations or conscious deception. This impression seemed to be substantiated by five normal electroencephalograms. However, when the electroencephalogram was taken in light sleep, the typical negative spike in the left anterior temporal area with phase reversal in other leads was elicited. The same pattern was obtained in a second record taken in light sleep and thus the diagnosis of psychomotor epilepsy was established.

The episodes of automatic disorganized behavior without loss of consciousness presents a diagnostic problem of greater magnitude than the first group. This is due to the following: loss of awareness during a seizure is believed by many to be a prerequisite for the diagnosis of epilepsy; the seizures in question may be of longer duration than the classical types, and the behavior is more coordinated and directed toward a goal than in the typical psychomotor attacks; the seizure in question may simulate emotional outbursts, due purely to psychogenic causes; affective changes such as depression may precede the acute attacks by periods of days. These episodes were known to the older observers in the preelectroencephalogram era under the name of hystero-epilepsy and affect-epilepsy. The reader is referred to an exhaustive review of hystero-epilepsy and affect-epilepsy by Notkin.[10] Cases reviewed by Notkin convey the impression, however, that the older authors also included in this category psychomotor attacks, cases of conversion hysteria, as well as cases under discussion. In spite of the limitations of electroencephalography, it has greatly contributed to the study of this type of case.

Waggoner and Bacchi[11] described, under paroxysmal convulsive disorder, variants of this, such as patients with attacks of dizziness, headache, unreasonable anger, assaultive behavior and abdominal discomfort. These patients had abnormal electroencephalographic tracings and improved with anticonvulsive medication. Gibbs and Gibbs[12,13] isolated, under the name of thalamic and hypothalamic epilepsy, paroxysmal behavior disorders characterized by rage reactions, weeping, and frequent autonomic phenomena such as palpitations and flushing. Their behavior is directed toward a goal and consciousness is preserved. The electroencephalogram shows a rather characteristic pattern consisting of bilateral, but not synchronous, 6 and 14 per second positive temporal spikes.

Case 3

A. P., a 32-year-old male, was referred for depression and irritability ending with destructive behavior. His history included enuresis until the age of ten, and a homosexual assault upon him when he was six years old. A. D. enlisted in the Army in 1940 and was discharged in 1947 at the rank of corporal. He married in 1946, after a six-month courtship, and he has been a good provider, a good husband, and a good father, except for the episodes of affective changes and destructive behavior. His first attack was in 1947, and all subsequent attacks, which have been occurring two to three times a year, followed the same pattern. In the beginning, the patient becomes depressed, moody, and irritable. He feels that his wife is picking on him and is too critical of his activities. He loses his appetite and prefers to stay by himself. He experiences a progressive increase of inner tension for a period of one week, and then he has a feeling of an "explosion" in the epigastrium and a feeling of bursting blood vessels. This is followed by a sudden outburst of violence such as smashing windows, hitting his head against the wall, etc. After approximately thirty minutes, the patient quiets down. For a few days following the destructive outburst, he complains of general malaise and nervousness.

Physicians who saw him during the acute phase of the attack could converse with him and, in general, had the impression that his awareness was not impaired. The patient was able to remember his attacks, including the acute phase. A purely psychogenic condition was suspected and this impression was reinforced by a history of enuresis, homosexual assault upon him, and so forth. The electroencephalogram, however, showed nonsynchronous 6 per second positive spikes in the midtemporal and posterior temporal regions on either side. Although the 14 per second positive spikes were not observed, the diagnosis was thalamic and hypothalamic epilepsy and the patient was treated with anticonvulsive medication.

Case 4

J. E., age 31, had no difficulties and made an excellent adjustment until 1944, when his ship received a direct hit by an enemy torpedo and he was stunned and thrown 15 feet away from the place where he had been standing. Following this experience, he became irritable and intolerant of noise. Upon his evacuation to the United States, he felt he could no longer control his emotions and he cried easily at the slightest provocation. He developed an urge to smash things and scream. Once, while in a hotel room, he developed an attack of rage and violence, during which he pulled hair out of his head, smashed the walls and it took four people to restrain him. He never had a recollection of the episode. He was discharged from the navy in 1945 with the diagnosis, "no disease found." Later, however, the Veterans Administration awarded him 50 per cent disability and he was given a diagnosis of anxiety state. Since he made a poor adjustment to civilian life, he enlisted in the Army in 1947. During his two years of enlistment he was frequently tense, restless, and finally obtained, not a disability but a dependency discharge.

Since his discharge from the Army in 1949, he has had attacks of irrepressible anger and long fugue states during which he left home and led an aimless, nomadic existence for several months. In addition to these symptoms, he developed attacks of violence, two to three times a year. Each attack was preceded by irritability, withdrawal, fear of getting into an argument, headaches starting in the back of his neck and spreading to the scalp, crying spells, a feeling of being "no good, fouled up, and there is nothing I can do about it." After approximately one week of feeling that way, he suddenly became extremely violent, smashing windows and dishes, but throughout his violence, the awareness of his environment is preserved. The attack ends with a feeling of guilt and suicidal thoughts. In addition to the attacks of violence, the patient had experienced occasional "fainting spells" without convulsions, and sudden, uncontrollable and unprovoked attacks of weeping. An episode of depression lasting a few days follows an attack of weeping. Between attacks the patient is able to work and support his family.

Since his electroencephalogram, taken on several occasions, showed bursts of irregular hypersynchronous waves and diffuse spikes, and sharp waves in addition to negative spikes in the left midtemporal and posterior temporal regions, with phase reversal in other leads, it became obvious that he had a variety of psychic seizures and was given an anticonvulsive medication. Shortly after treatment, he spontaneously reported that his nightmares had disappeared. He had a few typical psychomotor attacks with loss of consciousness in the beginning, but later all of his attacks had characteristics similar to those described in Case 3, except that the electroencephalogram did not show the characteristic pattern described by Gibbs in hypothalamic epilepsy.

PHENOMENA RELATED TO THE AUTONOMIC NERVOUS SYSTEM

Gowers,[14] in 1907, described under the name "borderland of epilepsy" various paroxysmal disturbances such as attacks of vertigo, fainting spells, and vaso-vagal attacks. Under vaso-vagal attacks, he meant paroxysms of tachycardia, feelings of suffocation, nausea, hot and cold flushes, and sweating and shivering accompanied by fear and agony. Penfield,[15] in 1929, described under the name diencephalic epilepsy, attacks of flushing of the face, sweating, lacrimation, salivation, gooseflesh, shivering, and a rise in blood pressure in a patient with a tumor compressing the anterior thalamic nuclei. In Wilson's[16] textbook of neurology, similar phenomena are described under the name "periventricular epilepsy," since it was felt that the "excessive neuronal discharge" took place in the nuclei of the fourth ventricle. It is, however, interesting to note that in Wilson's case, after the termination of the attack, "an overpowering nightmare of depression seized the patient, making him feel frankly suicidal."

It is quite obvious that attacks of hyperactivity of the autonomic centers have been described under various names by earlier authors, and it is also obvious that these attacks were known to be connected frequently with affective changes. The dramatic phenomena described in these cases are also observed during attacks of anxiety. Since anxiety neurosis is of much more frequent occurrence than the autonomic epilepsies, it is to be expected that the latter will be misdiagnosed and treated as a purely psychiatric condition.

Case 5

S. G., a 28-year old male, first developed symptoms in 1949 shortly after the accidental death of his brother. One day, while at work in the garage where he was employed as auto mechanic, he passed bloody urine. Shortly afterwards, he experienced faintness, a feeling of impending doom and perspired profusely. The attack lasted just a few minutes, but the employer urged him to see a doctor, who found a temperature of 101 degrees Fahrenheit and gave him penicillin. Since then, he has had rather frequent attacks consisting of an ill-described sensation in the occipital region and neck, general haziness of consciousness, goose pimples, cold and clammy extremities, rapid heartbeat, and a feeling of bloating and shrinking in the epigastrium. The attacks are occasionally preceded by flushing of the face and neck, which may be noticed by observers and is experienced by the patient as a burning sensation. A day or two before an attack, the patient may feel restless and aggressive, but after the attack there is a feeling of depression and despondency lasting for two to three days. Independent of the attacks described above, the patient had experienced a compulsion to harm somebody with his dead brother's knife. The feeing creeps up on him for a day or two, during which time he tries to fight it off, and on one occasion he even threw the knife out. His past history shows that he was shot through the chest during the war and a year before the first attack he sustained a brain concussion.

The patient's attacks have dramatically improved with Dilantin. He was free of attacks for a period of four months when he decided to stop taking the medication. The symptoms returned shortly afterwards. He previously carried the diagnosis of anxiety neurosis, but psychotherapy administered for a year previously failed to improve his symptoms. The electroencephalogram was conspicuously abnormal. There were long runs of flat top 5 per second waves with 6 per second positive spikes, particularly prominent in the right temporal area, and more pronounced during and after hyperventilation.

AKINETIC SEIZURES

Akinetic seizures consist of sudden loss of postural control, during which the patientcollapses, falling to the floor. Lennox[7] included the akinetic seizures in the petit mal triad. However, the 3 per second wave spike complex is not as characteristic, and drugs of the oxazolidin group are not as specific for akinetic seizures as for the two other members of the triad (myoclonic seizures and absence of pyknolepsy). The myoclonic epilepsy and absence are always genetic, whereas akinetic seizures may be due to subtentorial lesions, encephalitis, and ischemia of the brain stem. The clinical manifestations may be confused with cataplexy, syncope, or conversion hysteria. The catalectic attack, however, should be eliminated on clinical grounds, since it occurs during an emotional stimulus, such as laughter, and is usually associated with narcolepsy. The cause of syncope should be sought through various tests, such as carotid sinus stimulation, 5 hour sugar tolerance test (a 2 or 3 hour sugar tolerance test may be misleading, since the curve may reach hypoglycemic level in the 4th or 5th hour only) and studies for cardiac disease, variations of blood pressure, and so forth. The reader is referred for a detailed discussion of syncope to the monograph by Engel.[17] Electroencephalography, in spite of its limitations, may be a very valuable diagnostic tool, particularly if the 3 per second wave spike complex is elicited.

Case 6

N. A., a 32-year-old male, was in a good general physical condition until July, 1952 when his left hand was mutilated by the propeller of an onrushing plane. A month later, while bending down to shine his shoes, he suddenly experienced a feeling of light-headedness and fell down on his face. He remained unconscious for several minutes and was taken to an army hospital, where the doctor told him that he suffered from "worries" and "shock." Since that time, however, he has had two to three short similar attacks a year. There was a history of convulsions in infancy; otherwise, the past medical history is noncontributory. When examined, his neurologic and physical examinations were negative, carotid sinus test and 5 hour sugar tolerance test were also normal. Conversion hysteria was suspected and a battery of projective tests seemed to point in this direction. This was accepted as the diagnosis, particularly when several routine electroencephalograms showed a perfectly normal tracing. However, in light to moderate sleep induced by 0.2 gram (gr. 3) of seconal orally, a very typical 3 per second wave spike complex was elicited in all the leads. The sleep electroencephalogram was repeated on three different occasions and each time a similar pattern was obtained. The diagnosis was changed then to akinetic epilepsy.

COMMENT AND SUMMARY

It was obvious, even to the earlier investigators, that not all epileptic phenomena can be fitted into the three classical types, and that typical seizures may be modified to such an extent that they may pass unrecognized. Paroxysmal phenomena involving the activity of the autonomic nervous system, psychic functions, or both, as well as akinetic attacks, are at times serious problems in differentiation from purely psychiatric conditions. Electroencephalography as a diagnostic tool has its limitations, since epileptic-like activity can be found in nonepileptics and, on the other hand, normal interseizure electroencephalograms are found in some epileptics. In some instances, however, the electroencephalogram does not yield satisfactory results because only routine records are taken, without the benefit of activation methods such as sleep. Of the 6 cases presented in this paper, cases two and six had normal routine electroencephalograms on several occasions. Yet, in sleep, a typical psychomotor pattern was found in Case 2, and a 3 per second wave-spike pattern characteristic for petit mal triad in Case 6. A combination of autonomic and psychic phenomena is frequent, and there are apparently many transitional forms with quantitative differences. Thus, the patient in Case 1, during auras, referring to a temporal focus discharge, experienced pilo-erection. Case 5, whose autonomic phenomena were prominent, experienced a feeling of depression before and after the attack and, in addition, had episodes of obsessive thinking.

In the seizures characterized purely by psychic phenomena, various transitional forms, between cases with complete dissolution of consciousness and relative preservation of consciousness, are found. Case 4, for instance, experienced seizures with complete dissolution of consciousness and also with relative preservation of awareness and memory. Whether the affective changes preceding and following the attack should be considered as part of the seizure, or purely psychogenic manifestations, can be disputed. However, there constancy, order of occurrence, and relief by anticonvulsive medication seems to point to the former.

REFERENCES

1. Gibbs, F. A., Gibbs, L. A., & Lennox, W. G. (1943). Electroencephalographic classification of epileptics and controls. *Arc Neurol & Psychiat, 50*:111.
2. Abbott, J. H., & Schwab, R. S. (1946). Normal electroencephalograms in patients having proven epilepsy. *Nerv & Ment Dis, 26*:332.
3. Ostow, M., & Ostow, M. (1946). Paroxysmal slow activity in the electroencephalograms of non-epileptics. *J Nerv & Ment Dis, 103*:346.
4. Silverman, D. (1943). Clinical and electroencephalographic studies on clinical psychopaths. *Arch Neurol & Psychiat, 50*:18.
5. Cattell, J. P. & Pacella, B. L. (1950). Electroencephalographic and clinical study of children with primary behavior disorders. *Am J Psychiat, 107*: 25.
6. Clark, D. S. & Taylor, F. H. (1949). Clinical and electroencephalographic studies of prisoners charged with murder. *J Neurol Neurosurg & Psychiat, 12*:325.
7. Lennox, W. (1945). The petit mal epilepsies – Their treatment with Tridione. *J.A.M.A., 129*:1069.
8. Antoni, N. (1946). Dreamy states, epileptic aura, depersonalization and psychaesthenic fits. *Acta Psychiat et Neurol, 21*:1.
9. Gibbs, E. L., Gibbs, F. A. & Fuster, B. (1948). Psychomotor epilepsy. *Arch Neurol & Psychiat, 60*:331.
10. Notkin, J. (1930) "Affect epilepsy" and "hystero-epilepsy" A study of convulsive states in psychopaths. *J Nerv & Ment Dis, 72*:135.
11. Waggoner, R. W. & Bacchi, B. K. (1946). Paroxysmal convulsive disorder variants. *Proc A Res Nerv & Ment Dis, 26*:328.
12. Gibbs, E. L. & Gibbs, F. A. (1951). Electroencephalographic evidence of tha lamic and hypothalamic epilepsy. *Neurology, 1*:136.
13. Gibbs, F. A. & Gibbs, E. L. (1952). *Atlas of Electroencephalography*, Vol 2. pp. 329-346. Cambridge, MA: Addison and Wesley Press, Inc.
14. Gowers, W. R. (1907). *The borderland of epilepsy.* London: G. A. Churchill, Inc.
15. Penfield, W. (1929). Diencephalic autonomic epilepsy. *Arch Neurol & Psychiat, 22*:358.
16. Wilson, S. A. K. (1940). *Neurology, Vol. 2.* Baltimore: Williams and Wilkins Co.
17. Engel, G. L. (1950). *Fainting–Physiological and psychological correlations.* Springfield, IL: Charles C Thomas.

Chapter 16

DIAGNOSTIC PROBLEMS IN EPILEPSY

For euphemistic purposes, epilepsy is frequently presented under the heading of convulsive disorders. This, however, is a misnomer, since convulsions are characteristic only for the variety known as grand mal epilepsy. There is an array of epileptic phenomena manifested either by attacks of loss of consciousness as a sole symptom, or by motor, sensory, autonomic and psychic paroxysms with or without loss of consciousness.

Epilepsy comes from a Greek word meaning seizure. The ancients thoughts that an epileptic paroxysm was due to intervention of supernatural causes such as deities or evil spirits. Hippocrates, in his treatise on the "Sacred Disease," denounced the concept of supernatural causation of epilepsy by saying, "It arises like other disease–from things which enter and quit the body, such as cold, sun and the winds; things which are ever-changing and never at rest." Hughlings Jackson, at the end of the last century, introduced the concept of the epileptic paroxysm as being a clinical expression of an excessive neuronal discharge in the brain. This concept was further verified by the introduction of clinical electroencephalography in the early 1930s. Later bioelectric studies on experimental animals, as well as the result of Penfield's studies on brains of patients during surgical removal of epileptogenic foci, leave no doubt that Hughlings Jackson was correct. Thus, it is now universally accepted that an epileptic paroxysm is a clinical correlation of excessive bioelectric activity in the brain. The clinical picture of the seizure depends on the focus, intensity and spread of the discharge.

Methods of Diagnosis. Every paroxysmal disorder may be sus-

Source: Revitch, E. (1956). Diagnostic problems in epilepsy. *Medical Times: The Journal of General Practice, 84*:1056-1065.

pected of being a clinical expression of an excessive neuronal discharge, i.e., a form of epilepsy. The diagnosis should be made on the basis of a very thorough anamnesis, neurological and psychiatric examination, and electroencephalography.

A. Of all the three steps, the thorough history taking, with a scrupulous recording of the seizure, is by far the most important. The initial phenomena of the seizure, which in essence are the clinical expressions of the physiological events at the discharging focus, remain too frequently unrecorded by nurses and physicians. Yet, these initial phenomena, as well as the progression of the events, are frequently the sole diagnostic clue that the paroxysm is an epileptic, and not a psychogenic, manifestation.

The initial phenomena may be divided into (a) motor, (b) sensory, (c) visceral, and (d) psychic. The motor phenomena may consist of Jacksonian seizures and adversive movements. The Jacksonian seizure is manifested by unilateral involvement which may or may not spread to the opposite side. A complete knowledge of brain anatomy is necessary to understand the succession of events in a Jacksonian seizure. In general, the Jacksonian motor seizures indicate a lesion of the contralateral motor strip. Adversive movements consist of slow rotation of the head to one side. This indicates a contralateral lesion in the premotor area.

Initial sensory, visceral, and psychic manifestations of a seizure are commonly known as aura. The sensory aura may consist either of various parethesias involving one side of the body, or of visual, auditory and olfactory hallucinations. In the case of parethesias, one must suspect a lesion in the contralateral parietal lobe. In the case of hallucinations, the involvement of the temporal lobe on either side is in question. However, in the case of visual hallucinations as initial phenomena of a seizure, one must distinguish the formed from the unformed hallucinations. Formed hallucinations (visions of animate or inanimate objects) indicate that the lesion is located in the posterior portion of the temporal lobe on either side, while unformed visual hallucinations, such as flashes of light, dots, spots, and so forth. indicate an occipital focus.

Epigastric sensations according to Penfield and Kristiansen[1] are connected with a focus in the temporal lobe, sylvian fissure, or in the region of insula. Autonomic and psychic phenomena (gooseflesh, flushing, anxiety, etc.) are also indicative of a temporal focus. For a more complete study of the initial phenomena, the reader is referred to Penfield and Kristiansen.[1] In addition to initial phenomena, a postictal event called Todd's paralysis is frequently an important diagnostic clue as far as the focus of the seizure is concerned. Todd's paralysis consists of a short weakness or paralysis of a limb, contralateral to the discharging focus, during the post-ictal recovery. To illustrate the importance of initial phenomena and of a thorough history-taking, the following case is presented.

Case 1

A 32-year-old male was admitted to the hospital for attacks of falling down, rolling on the floor with aimless flailing of the extremities and fighting those who approached him. Since several EEG's were negative and the seizures atypical, he was diagnosed on previous admissions as psychopathic personality and schizophrenia. A thorough anamnesis, however, elicited mounting epigastric sensations and a formed visual hallucination (a candle surrounded by a halo) preceding the events described above. Additional electroencephalograms taken in sleep then elicited a focus in the left temporal region, thus substantiating the epileptic rather than the psychogenic nature of the disorder. In this case, the presence of an epigastric and visual aura, not elicited at the previous examinations, made the diagnosis of epilepsy certain. Electroencephalography substantiated the diagnosis but it was the thorough anamnesis which made it clear.

B. A neurological, and frequently a psychiatric, examination is necessary in all cases of seizures; although, in most instances even with a definite focal pattern, no abnormal neurological signs will be found. Even in cases caused by tumors, the neurological examination may remain negative for a long time. The question whether air studies should be done in all cases of focal seizures (i.e., seizures which start with initial motor or sensory phenomena thus indicating a focus of discharge) cannot be answered with certainty. It is obvious that hospitalized patients will undergo air studies more often than out-patients. In office practice, it is also obvious that a neurosurgeon will recur to air studies more readily than a general neuropsychiatrist. It was shown, however, that in cases of brain tumors, air studies do not yield positive results when the neurological examination is negative.[2]

C. Electroencephalography is indispensable as a diagnostic tool. An epileptic clinic without electroencephalographic facilities is an anachronism at the present time. Yet, electroencephalography is only a diagnostic tool supplementing clinical findings and not the procedure making the diagnosis. It is perhaps more important for the referring physician to know the limitations of electroencephalography than its potentialities. Thus, the methods of recording, labeling, and the placement of electrodes vary with various workers. Therefore, it may be difficult for the electroencephalographer to pronounce himself on a record taken in a different laboratory. The electroencephalography is not as well standardized as electrocardiography, therefore, one encounters many so-called borderline records. Artefacts are frequent and, at times, cannot be readily distinguished from brain waves. It is estimated by some observers that about 20 percent of interseizure records are negative.[3] In my opinion, this is a very conservative estimate. One routine record may show no abnormalities and the EEG may become abnormal with various methods of activation such as sleep and slow I.V. injection of Metrazol. Thus, in Case 1 presented here, numerous records were negative, but yielded positive results in light sleep. EEG patterns in children are less regular and slower than in adults.

Interpretation of EEG's in childhood presents many difficulties and requires special experience in tracings with the younger age group. All this shows the difficulties of the EEG and the fallacies of final statements after only one recording, as is often done in office practice. A practitioner not well-versed in epileptology and not approximately acquainted with the fundamentals of the EEG will do better in referring his or her patient for a consultation, leaving up to the consultant what diagnostic methods to use.

DIAGNOSTIC PROBLEMS

Brain Tumors. Seizures starting with an aura, or initial motor phenomena, indicate a focal discharge spreading to the other areas of the brain. Penfield[4] classifies all these seizures as focal seizures. The lesions found at the discharging foci are the following, according to Penfield: (a) brain tumor, (b) cerebral cicatrix, (c) local cerebral atrophy, (d) local microgeria, and (e) brain cyst.

Of all these lesions, the brain tumor is of the greatest importance. Seizures are more commonly associated with the slowly growing benign tumors than with the rapidly growing malignant tumors. According to Penfield and Jasper (4), 40 percent of all patients who had seizures, secondary to brain tumors, had them as their initial symptom. A physician should be particularly alert and suspicious when the first seizure occurs in an adult.

Febrile Seizures. Convulsions associated with fever in children under the age of five years are not uncommon. A question arises as to whether they indicate a predisposition to seizures, or if they should be considered as benign events without further consequence. Lennox[5] quotes Thom and Wegman as saying that a history of an early infantile convulsion is obtained in 20 percent to 50 percent of adult epileptics. Lennox[5] concludes that febrile convulsions may presage recurrent seizures in the future, if the first convulsion occurs before the age of one year (and after the age of 3 years), when convulsions are frequent, when birth is abnormal, when there is epilepsy in the family, and the EEG is abnormal. Schmidt and Ward[5], in their review of the literature, show a variety of opinions. They, however, agree essentially with the conclusions of Lennox.[5]

Petit Mal and Minor Seizures. Many physicians, perhaps the majority, label as petit mal all the minor seizures which are not characterized by a major convulsion. This is erroneous, not only from a purely academic but also from a practical therapeutic viewpoint. True petit mal seizures respond to the oxazolidine Dione group or drugs [Tridione,[7] Paradione[8]] and to Milontin,[9] while the other types of seizures may be aggravated. To the contrary, the drugs which are employed in the treatment of grand mal seizures (Dilantin,[10] Mesantoin,[11] Mysoline,[12]) may aggravate the true petit mal. The true petit mal seizures are characterized by their greater frequency in children than in adults, by the short duration of each paroxysm, and by the frequency of the attacks. Ten to 20 attacks a day is not too uncommon. The electroencephalographic findings are typical and consist of the characteristic spike 3-5 per second wave complexes. The characteristic tracing, however, may be obtained only during and after hyperventilation and with activation methods such as slow I.V. injection of Metrazol, sleep, or photic stimulation. Thus, an EEG without the typical petit mal pattern does not absolutely rule out petit mal.

Lennox[13] demonstrated three types of petit mal seizures which he grouped under the name of petit mal triad: (1) petit mal absence of pyknolepsy (which consists in transient loss of consciousness lasting only a few seconds and which is clinically manifested by pallor and short staring spells), (2) myoclonic epilepsy (not to be confused with myoclonus epilepsy of Unverricht) which is characterized by a few myoclonic twitches of extremities and eyelids with loss of consciousness lasting only a few seconds, and (3) akinetic epilepsy which is characterized by collapse of muscle tone and falling down, with a brief loss of consciousness.

The minor seizures, so frequently confused with petit mal attacks, are usually aborted major seizures. The course of the seizure is curtailed either by administration of drugs or by other factors such as an insufficiently strong discharge. Very often the seizure may be reduced to the initial motor phenomena or to the aura. Thus, the whole paroxysm may consist of an adversive movement, numbness of the extremities contralateral to the lesion, and epigastric discomfort in case of a focus in the temporal lobe or in the region of insula. The staring spells in temporal lobe foci are frequently diagnosed as petit mal seizures. A thorough scrutiny however, would reveal in these patients epigastric sensations preceding the seizure and frequency of epigastric sensations without any other evidence of an attack. The following case history will illustrate the misdiagnosis of staring spells as petit mal seizures.

Case 2

A 16-year-old boy developed staring spells of short duration, during which the head was turned to the right side, skin was pale and covered with goose pimples. The patient also claimed that some of the seizures were induced by thinking of various events in the past, for instance the camp where he spent a summer. The EEG showed a focus in the left temporal area. The autonomic phenomena, and the inducement of a seizure through memory mechanisms, is known in epileptic discharges originating in the temporal lobe. The rotation of the head to the right indicated, on purely clinical grounds, that the focus was on the left side. Tridione administered by his physician only aggravated the condition, while administration of Dilantin and Phenobarbital reduced the number of the seizures to a minimum.

Case 3

A 6-year-old girl developed attacks of staring spells lasting about 5 minutes. These were frequently preceded by abdominal complaints. In addition, she had abdominal complaints, without staring spells, diagnosed as G.I. upsets.

In true petit mal absences, there are no initial motor or sensory phenomena and the attacks are of much shorter duration than in the two preceding cases.

Abdominal Symptoms in Epilepsy. Epigastric sensations, as an initial phenomenon in seizures, were alluded to previously in this paper. Penfield[1,4] found the discharging focus to be located in the sylvian fissure, insula, or temporal lobe. Epigastric sensations without a fully developed seizure are frequent and, at times, misdiagnosed as gastro-intestinal upsets. Moore[14-16] described an entity he named abdominal epilepsy. This is characterized by paroxysmal abdominal pain and abnormal electroencephalograms. The attacks of abdominal pain may be accompanied by nausea and vomiting and may terminate with general achiness and sleep. Many of Moore's cases, as well as cases of authors cited by him, had a history of head injury, brain tumor, and post-infectious encephalopathies. The focal lesion causing the seizures is thought to be in Brodman areas 6, 5, 3 (in the frontal and parietal lobes). In one of Moore's cases,[16] the extirpation of a brain tumor in area 6 cured the paroxysmal abdominal pain.

Paroxysmal Phenomena with Psychiatric Implications. The physician may frequently be called to decide whether attacks of unconsciousness, unusual motor phenomena, autonomic discharges, and paroxysmal behavioral abnormalities are psychogenic manifestations or of epileptic origin. As indicated in a previous publication,[17] only a thorough knowledge of psychiatric diagnoses, of the initial phenomena of seizures, and of the value and limitations of electroencephalography will make such a diagnosis possible. There are no rules of the thumb for such a differentiation; however, a few basic data on what was previously called epileptic equivalents, as well as on autonomic epilepsy, is necessary.

The so-called epileptic equivalents of the pre-EEG era are now usually described under the term psychomotor epilepsy. A few years ago Gibbs and Gibbs[18] added to the family of epileptic equivalents, thalamic and hypothalamic epilepsy. Psychomotor epilepsy is chiefly characterized by attacks of behavioral disorganization with loss of consciousness. The paroxysm may be of a rather simple pattern, such as smacking of the lips and repetitive aimless movements, or it may consist of more complex patterns such as fugues, attacks of furor, and assaultiveness. The patient is not conscious of his environment and the whole attack is covered with amnesia. Most, but not all of the attacks of psychomotor epilepsy, are connected with a focus in the temporal lobe. The paroxysms therefore may start with olfactory hallucinations (the so-called uncinate fits), formed visual hallucinations, or visual disturbances such as macropsia and micropsia. Epigastric sensations as an initial phenomenon of the seizure are extremely common. A negative spike in the anterior temporal region was demonstrated in psychomotor epilepsy by Gibbs, Gibbs and Fuster[19]. However, the typical tracing will not be obtained in all cases of psychomotor epilepsy; furthermore, the characteristic spike may be elicited in sleep only. Psychomotor epilepsy is known to show, in the interval of seizures, an unstable behavior pattern and psychic abnormalities, at times of psychotic proportions.

Case 4

A 27-year-old male developed sudden outbursts of assaultiveness and furor lasting for one half hour. There was a complete amnesia for the outbursts. In between the paroxysms, the patient experienced vague paranoid delusions and auditory and visual hallucinations. An EEG showed a negative sharp wave in the right anterior temporal region.

Thalamic and hypothalamic epilepsy is characterized by a specific electroencephalogram (6 and 14 per second positive spikes). The clinical manifestations consist of rage reactions, weeping, and autonomic phenomena such as palpitations and flushing of the face. Consciousness during the paroxysm is at least partially preserved.

Case 5

A 32-year-old male has been having attacks of rage and destructiveness preceded by depression for a period of approximately one week. Immediately prior to the attack, he experienced epigastric distress. After 15 minutes to one-half hour of rage, he feels rather well and is able to function up to the next attack. Consciousness though hazy, and memory of the attack, are preserved. An EEG showed six per second positive sharp waves (no 14 per second waves could be elicited).

Autonomic seizures were described in 1907 by Gowers 20 under the name of vaso-vagal attacks. These attacks consisted of tachycardia, feelings of suffocation, nausea, hot and cold flashes, pallor, sweating, shivering, fear, and agony. In 1929, Penfield 21 described similar attacks, under the name of diencephalic epilepsy, in a patient with a brain tumor compressing the anterior thalamic nuclei. A case reported previously[22] will serve as an illustration of autonomic seizures.

Case 6

A 28-year-old male had attacks of haziness of consciousness, goose pimples, tachycardia, a feeling of bloating, and shrinking in the epigastrium, as well as anxiety and a feeling of impending death. After the termination of the attack, he remained depressed for several days. EEG tracings consisted of 5 per second flat top waves in the right midtemporal region. He markedly improved with anticonvulsive medication. For a year prior to the examination, he was successfully treated in a mental hygiene clinic with psychotherapy for anxiety neurosis.

In connection with this case, it is interesting to note that Wilson[23] described, in his textbook, depression following an autonomic attack. Paroxysmal psychiatric manifestations with hyperventilation, fainting spells, autonomic reactions, or outbursts of blind rage are constantly a source of diagnostic difficulties. The diagnostic problem is complicated by borderline or abnormal EEG's which are quite frequent in children with behavior disorders,[24] and were also described by various authors in prison inmates,[25,26] and in the so-called aggressive psychopaths.[27] It is not unusual to find patients of this type misdiagnosed as epileptic and treated with anticonvulsive medication. On the other hand, it has also been my experience that psychomotor epileptics were misdiagnosed as psychopathic personality or schizophrenia, due to interseizure personality deviations which were so prominent that the paroxysmal epileptic manifestations passed unnoticed.[28]

SUMMARY

Thorough history taking, knowledge of the initial phenomena of seizures and, in some cases, of psychiatric diagnosis, are essential in dealing with diagnostic problems in epilepsy. Electroencephalography is a useful laboratory tool but it is not as well standardized as electrocardiography; therefore, it should not be used blindly as a "shot gun" diagnostic procedure. Attention was paid to the distinction between true petit mal and minor, aborted seizures, and the therapeutic significance of this distinction was stressed. A short description of seizures connected with brain tumors, fever, abdominal epilepsy, and of seizures with psychiatric implications was given.

REFERENCES

1. Penfield, W., & Kristiansen, K. (1951). *Epileptic seizure patterns.* Springfield, IL: Charles C Thomas,
2. Martin, H. L. & McDowell, F. (1954). Evaluation of seizures in the adult. *Arch Neurol Psychiat, 71*:101.
3. Abbott, J. H. & Schwab, R. S. (1948). Normal electroencephalogram in patients having proven epilepsy. *Proc A. Res Nerv Ment Dis, 26*:332.
4. Penfield, W. & Jasper, H. (1954). Epilepsy and the functional anatomy of the human brain. Boston: Little Brown and Company.
5. Lennox, M. (1946). Febrile convulsions in childhood. *Proc. An Res Nerv Ment Dis, 26*:342.
6. Schmidt, R. P. & Ward, A. A. Jr. (1955). Febrile convulsions. *Epilepsia, 4*:41.
7. Tridione-Trimethadione (Abbott).
8. Paradione-Dimethyl-ethyl-oxazlidine-dione (Abbott).
9. Milontin-Methyl-phenyl-Succinamide (Parke-Davis).
10. Dilantin-Diphenyl-hydantoin-sodium (Parke-Davis).
11. Mesantoin-Mathyl-phenyl-ethyl-hydantoin (Sandoz).
12. Mysoline-Brand of Primidone (Ayerst).
13. Lennox, W. G. (1945). The petit mal epilepsies: Their treatment with Tridione. *JAMA, 129*:1069.
14. Moore, M. T.(1944). Paroxysmal abdominal pain. A form of focal symptomatic epilepsy. *JAMA, 124*:561.
15. Moore, M. T. (1950). Abdominal epilepsy. *Am Med Sc, 220*:87.
16. Moore, M. T. (1950). Epilepsie abdominale. *Journal Suisse de Medicine, 80*:1352.
17. Revitch, E. (1955). Psychiatric aspects of epilepsy. *Journ Med Soc New Jersey, 52*:634.
18. Gibbs, E. L. & Gibbs, F. A. (1951). Electroencephalographic evidence of thalamic and hypothalamic epilepsy. *Neurology, 1*:136.
19. Gibbs, E. L., Gibbs, F. A., & Fuster, B. (1948). Psychomotor epilepsy. *Arch Neurol Psychiat, 60*:331.
20. Gowers, W. R. (1907). The borderland of epilepsy. London: B. A. Churchill, Inc.
21. Penfield, W. (1929). Diencephalic autonomic epilepsy. *Arch Neurol Psychiat, 22*:358.
22. Revitch, E. (1954). Epileptic manifestations resembling psychiatric disorders. *Journ Med Soc, New Jersey, 51*:3.
23. Wilson, S. A. K. (1940). *Neurology Vol. 2.* Baltimore: Wilkins and Wilkins.

24. Teterka, J. H. & Katz, J. (1955). Study of correlations between electroencephalographic and psychological patterns in emotionally disturbed children. *Psychosomatic Medicine, 17*:62.
25. Silverman, D. (1943). Clinical and electroencephalographic studies on criminal psychopaths. *Arch Neurol Psychiat, 50*:18.
26. Clark, D. S. & Taylor F. H. (1949). Clinical and electroencephalographic studies of prisoners charged with murder. *J Neurol Neurosurg Psychiat, 12*:325.
27. Hill, D. (1944). Cerebral dysrythmia. Its significance in aggressive behavior. *Proc Roy Soc Med, 37*:317.
28. Revitch, E. & Luzzi, M. (1953). Electroencephalographic survey of a mental hospital with special reference to temporal lobe abnormalities. *Dis Nerv Syst, 14*: 331.

Chapter 17

PSYCHOMOTOR PAROXYSMS OF NONEPILEPTIC ORIGIN

Paroxysmal outbursts of disorganized behavior with or without hypermotility, autonomic manifestations, falling down, and various degrees of alterations of consciousness, frequently present a difficult problem in the differential diagnosis between epileptic and nonepileptic disorders. In accordance with the Jacksonian concept, we now believe that the clinical manifestations of epilepsy are correlates of an excessive neuronal discharge in the brain. Unfortunately, scalp electroencephalography is not always a reliable diagnostic tool since paroxysmal tracings may be found in nonepileptics, while perfectly normal records are not uncommon in epileptics. Furthermore, the very boundaries of epilepsy are not clear in spite of tremendous advances in the field. Thus, for instance, Schwade and Geiger[1] recently challenged the very concept of thalamic and hypothalamic epilepsy described by Gibbs and Gibbs.[2] According to the authors, the 6 and 14 second spikes described in this condition are connected not with epileptic phenomena, but with thalamic, hypothalamic and amygdalic impulses released by an emotional trigger.

H. Baruk and his school in France believe that, in addition to hysterical attacks, there is a whole spectrum of paroxysms extending from quasi-voluntary events to epileptic manifestations. The French authors have described these seizures under the name of "crises neuropathiques" and "crises catathymiques."[3,4] The views of the French authors seem to revive the old concept of Gowers[5] who questioned the existence of intermediate forms between hysteria and epilepsy.

Source: Revitch, E. (1958). Psychomotor paroxysms of non-epileptic origin. *Diseases of the Nervous System*, *19*:562-566.

For a period of over three years, I paid special attention to patients with paroxysmal psychic, motor, and autonomic phenomena which, at some time, were thought to be of epileptic origin and frequently treated as such with anticonvulsive medication. The clinical material was collected from inmates of the New Jersey prisons, among the cases referred to the New Jersey State Diagnostic Center by courts and agencies, and from patients with similar episodes seen in private practice. The institutional patients were particularly valuable since it was possible to observe them for two to three years and some of them were followed indirectly for a period of five years. This study, as well as a review of literature, clearly indicates a spectrum of conditions with various degrees of dominance of physiological and psychological factors in the causation of the seizures. It is possible to divide the attacks into four large and somewhat heterogeneous groups:

- Group 1. Physiological factors such as hypoglycemic reactions, syncopes, etc.
- Group 2. Attacks due to physiological and psychological factors with physiological dominance; these seizures are connected with physiological immaturity of the nervous tissue or to brain lesions. Due to this, emotionally triggered impulses cannot be coordinated into purposeful activity or inhibited. This is common in childhood encephalopathies, childhood schizophrenia, impulsive behavior connected with 6 and14 per second positive spikes, and in aggressive psychopaths with theta activity in the mid-temporal region as described by Hill.[6]
- Group 3. Physiological and psychological factors with psychological dominance: To this group belong outbursts of uncontrollable anxiety with behavioral disorganization, outbursts of anger, and excitement occasionally with breath-holding spells in paranoid personalities.
- Group 4. Due to psychological factors: To this group belong purely psychogenic conditions such as hysterical dissociations and simulation.

Most of the seizures observed by this author belong to Group 2 and 3. In Group 2, the most outstanding cause of diagnostic error were cases of childhood schizophrenia with various impulsive manifestations and blind rages. A thorough history taking usually revealed specific factors producing what would seem to be a psychomotor seizure. For instance, a three-year-old boy had attacks of uncontrollable rage, with falling down on the floor in specific situations such as men and women appearing together on television, his mother reading a newspaper, and so forth.

Group 3 was predominant among prison inmates of younger age groups. The seizures consisted in what seemed to be unprovoked rages with altercations of consciousness, assault, destruction of objects, self-destructiveness, as well as falling down or with disorganized purposeless motility. These attacks seemed so out of context that the patients received anticonvulsive medication prior to the re-evaluation of their condition. It appeared that practically all the subjects presenting with these phenomena were of a paranoid personality structure with a suspicious, distrustful, and hostile orientation to the human environment. At the New Jersey Reformatory for Women, 15 inmates with psychomotor outbursts were all classified as paranoid personality, while out of 20 inmates without psychomotor outbursts, and taken at random for this study, only four were classified as such. As a general rule, attacks in this group disappeared with emotional maturation, better motivation, and a supportive relationship with a member of the staff. EEG's were abnormal only in four out of 15 patients at the Reformatory for Women and were of borderline quality in a few other cases, in the younger age group, and normal in the majority of patients.

Many of the patients, in describing their seizures, brought up the subjective experience of bitemporal, throbbing headache, and difficulty in breathing prior to the blackout. Hypnosis, sodium amytal interviews, and repeated psychiatric examinations for a long period of time usually discovered precipitating incidents causing frustration and anger. Thus, a 28-year-old woman with a paranoid personality structure, who in adolescence was considered to have epileptic equivalents, described the attacks in her youth as follows: "I was depressed. I wanted to be with my mother. Nothing mattered. I was upset. It was mostly nerves but now I can control my temper." An inmate in a male prison presented attacks of falling down with loss of consciousness, as well as outbursts of blind range with assaultiveness. These attacks were provoked by quasi-delusional impressions that someone was going to hurt him. On a few occasions, he found himself in strange places, not knowing how he got there. On several occasions, when given sodium amytal intravenously, he became delirious, delusional, and dangerously assaultive. With a change of environment, and assignment to a shop with a sympathetic supervisor, the attacks disappeared in spite of removal of anticonvulsive medication. He had another attack, however, two years later when confronted with an unsympathetic individual who, he felt, wanted to harm him.

In the backgrounds of some individuals belonging to Group 2, occasional convulsive attacks can be elicited in the history. The case of a thirteen-year-old boy who had been followed for two years is a good example. He apparently had a convulsive seizure early in the morning at the age of eight and then at the age of 10 years. Repeated EEG's since the age of eight years revealed theta activity in the left temporal area. He was on anticonvulsive medication between the ages of 10 and 13 years, at which time, for a period of three weeks, he was tense, nervous, with attacks of flushing of the face, unprovoked assaults on his foster father and on his dog. An increase in anti-convulsive medication did not modify the pattern. During these three weeks, he was subject to severe emotional stress, since his mother planned to remove him from his foster parents whom he considered as his real parents. With a change of the stressful situation, the attacks disappeared and he has been free of any seizures for the past year, in spite of the fact that anticonvulsive medication had been withdrawn. The history of this boy and other similar cases bring forth the following hypothesis. A high threshold with epileptogenic focus may occasionally show up under strong stimuli. At the same time, the damaged area in the brain weakens the ability of the central nervous system to redirect or inhibit emotionally triggered release phenomena. This may also explain Gower's[5] assumption that some hysteroid seizures may later become real epileptic attacks.

DISCUSSION OF DOCTOR REVITCH'S PAPER

Doctor Hans Strauss: Doctor Revitch has presented much case material with a great variety of syndromes. He mentions, for example, hysterical dissociation, rage reactions, autonomic and psychic paroxysms. He has described akinetic seizures and breathholding spells without, however, adhering to the exact meaning which these words have in neuropsychiatric usage.

The characteristics common to all in Doctor Revitch's group is evidently the occurrence of short, episodic alterations of behavior which, in all his cases, appear in the background of less obvious chronic psychiatric difficulties. On the basis of these episodic disturbances, Doctor Revitch speaks of psychomotor paroxysms. He does not use the expressions psychomotor attack or psychomotor seizure. However, it seems to me that paroxysms, seizure, or attack signify essentially the same reaction and, therefore, as far as I can see, these patients do not suffer from what is generally called a psychomotor attack or seizure or paroxysm. The term psychomotor seizure, as it is now employed, following Gibbs and Lennox, is not well-chosen, for it denotes mainly those states which psychiatrists previously used to call twilight states or dreamy states. While I do not deny that such twilight states can occur outside the field of epilepsy, I do not see that the observations, made by Doctor Revitch, should be diagnosed as such states. Many of them show evidently an emotionally induced narrowing of consciousness, but no general depression of the level of consciousness. The word "psychomotor" should not be used to describe the conditions discussed by Doctor Revitch for this will inevitably lead to confusion and contribute nothing to the necessary clarification.

Is there any relationship between these cases and epilepsy? Of course, one will think of such a relationship in view of the episodic appearance of the disturbances. Many observations have been made, beginning with those of my teacher Kleist in 1926, up to those by Weil, Heath and Epstein, which have shown the importance of epileptic mechanism in some rather complicated episodic psychotic states. Doctor Revitch denies a relationship of his observations to epilepsy, on the basis of clinical and electroencephalographic studies. In most cases the EEG was normal, at least as long as no special provocative methods were used. In two cases, Doctor Revitch describes bursts of slow activity. Of course, this is an unspecific type of abnormality which is seen quite often in epilepsy but also in many other conditions.

However, the presence of this abnormality in these cases shows that they have a disturbance in cerebral activity which can be defined physiologically. This is, in my opinion, of the greatest importance. We should try in every psychiatric case to discover, by all available means, whether there is a disturbance of brain function which we can define in terms of brain physiology. Once we have found such a disturbance, the problem arises as to what is its role in the pathogenesis of the deviation in behavior. Are the psychiatric manifestations direct and simple, one might say obligatory, sequelae of the disturbed brain function as, for example, the appearance of photopsias with an irritative process in the optic system? If there are such obligatory sequelae, they will occur in every person with the same physiological disturbance of brain function, independent of personality make-up or the present situation. The relationship of the behavioral disorder to the disturbance of brain physiology may, however, be much more complicated. The abnormal cerebral activity may result primarily only in a slight diffuse disturbance of cerebral function. This disturbance, however, may make it impossible for the patient to cope with difficulties in the same way as a person without such a disturbance, and so lead to abnormal reactions whose type is determined by many factors including the personality of the patient, the present setting and others. In this respect, let me point out that probably quite a few of Doctor Revitch's patients suffered from some disturbance in cerebral physiology, even if their EEG was normal. Many of them had low IQ's pointing to some form of cerebral impairment.

I fully agree with the statement that there are patients with episodic outbursts of abnormal behavior in who no disturbance of brain physiology can be demonstrated by any means available now. Doctor Revitch would not have written this paper if he had not been fully aware of the fact that such a disturbance can be shown in others. Its demonstration is of theoretical and even practical importance. I refer here, as an example, only to those children with behavior disorders, and those psychopathic personalities who show bursts of slow activity in their EEG, and who can frequently be helped greatly by simple drug treatment.

While I have to disagree with many of Doctor Revitch's formulations, I feel that his paper is important because it brings up the problem of physiologically definable disturbances of brain activity in psychiatric disorders.

It is very gratifying to see, in the last years, how biological and physiological research begins to play an increasingly greater role in psychiatry. I am fully convinced that with the use of this approach and with the aid of new tools of research, (e.g. depth recording of the brain), we will, in the not too distant future, discover basic deviations of the brain from its normal physiological activity in conditions where such deviations were not even suspected before.

Doctor Leo Alexander: This is medically and legally a most important area, because in court cases these questions often arise, and those who have read Doctor Walter Lindsay Neustatter's book, *The Mind of the Murdered* (Christopher Johnson, London, 1957), may recall this. He also included a cause célèbre that we struggled with in Boston. Finally, Doctor Wm. G. Lennox was brought in as arbiter. In this case, a boy had killed his favorite aunt in a brutal attack, and the late Mr. Ogilvie called as technical consultant to the prison, at my suggestion, produced magnificent records of left temporal spikes. The boy had suffered a head injury, and his first convulsive seizure at age two, a second seizure and a fall down a flight of stairs at age 11. There were outbursts of brutal assaultiveness against playmates and siblings; once after an argument be put a plate of hot beans over the head of his brother, scalding him very severely. There were similar outbursts on three occasions with dysmnestic fugue states of varying duration while serving with the Marines, and the final brutal attack on the aunt. He had abnormal reflexes on the right, implicating the left pyramidal centers, and a definite left temporal lobe focus with spikes. I testified to that effect, but I was contradicted by a very venerable psychiatric expert, who stated that the EEG can never have any bearing on the mental state. He said he had seen many epileptics with very abnormal EEG's and yet were normal mentally, and seen brutal acts committed by people with normal EEG's. He claimed the abnormal EEG had no bearing at all.

I then testified that the temporal lobe focus, in view of Gibb's findings, has a certain specificity. Nevertheless, the jury convicted him because the venerable expert was more persuasive than my too scientific, too theoretical, testimony. Then a commission was appointed on which were epileptologists who confirmed my findings, did more electroencephalograms and the boy's sentence was commuted. When Doctor Walter Lindsay Neustatter came to Boston, I turned all the data over to him, which he included in his book. He reported some very interesting cases. From a medicolegal point of view, his problem is very important. Because if the person is an epileptic, there is a much stronger case.

Dennis Hill and William Sargant contributed an interesting case of matricide. This man killed his mother during the height of an argument in what appeared to be a psychomotor fit, facilitated by hyperventilation and hypoglycemia. The jury found him not guilty because of insanity.

Doctor Revitch's great contribution is that he brought to us clinical material that we rarely see except when brought into court. He sees it in pure culture in prison practice. The entire psychiatry of the criminal is virgin territory, never actually studied on a wide scale. I hope Doctor Revitch will make a systematic study because very little is really known about the subject.

In the Army, we saw many of this type. We saw many more of the things which you find rarely in civilian life. I don't know whether it is the pressure of Army life, the confinement, or what it is. The British made some statistical studies of the subject. More of those crimes occurred in cold weather than in hot weather. They thought that brain hydration had something to do with it.

Doctor Joachim Luwisch: I am inclined to agree with Doctor Straus. From Revitch's presentation, I am not convinced that those cases did not have epilepsy or a disorder which we call convulsive disorder.

I would like to ask Doctor Revitch, (a) did he try medications with those patients and did he see any change in their behavior, and (b) does he or did he take into consideration the fact that in about 5 per cent of proven cases the EEG is normal?

Doctor Leo Alexander: I agree with Doctor Luwisch that perhaps sleep recording may be in order in view of Gibbs' work.

Doctor Emerick Friedman: I would like to mention a classification of epileptic personality, somewhat in the discard at present, which contains references to phenomena that were described, namely, that various types of emotional outbursts can occur without definite EEG findings at the time or, let us say, that EEG's were not taken at the time of the events.

I have now several cases, referred by the New York State Rehabilitation Department, which has become interested in long term disabilities, in which certain phases of epilepsy have played a prominent role. Several instances have come up recently, in which the patients had a definite diagnosis of epilepsy and everyone who had seen these patients classified them as epileptic states.

In discussions with these patients, it was noted, between the attacks, the patients recognized and everybody around recognized, numerous outbursts of psychopathological phenomena, in some instances criminal psychopathology. No one took an EEG at the time. The patients were neither hysterical nor epileptic, presumably at that particular time. Is such a phenomenon of personality or of some other mechanism, some as yet undetermined type of electrophysiologic episode?

Doctor William Holt, Jr.: To me, the point of Doctor Revitch's paper is not that he had some people with epileptic EEG's and some with convulsions, but that he was dealing with a group in whom there often was found conscious awareness of their behavior during emotional outbursts or the outbursts of disordered behavior. In this respect, he considered them different than the classical hysterical patient and quite different from the classical epileptic patient. He saw that these were people, who had an unstable emotional make-up, with a tendency to get into antisocial activity and, of course, appeared primarily in prison populations.

I, also, see such patients occasionally and I think that Doctor Revitch has performed a useful service in pointing up the fact, that though there is some similarity between the epileptic and hysteric in these groups, in many instances, they are neither one nor the other. I think it would be well to exclude those that have definite epileptic histories or hysterical episodes so that we can focus more definitely on this intermediate group who very often are antagonistic and suspicious of people in general, especially authoritative figures

Doctor Leo Alexander: Doctor Holt has made a very important point and I would like to ask Doctor Revitch whether he has seen in his prison population any attempted suicides by impulsive individuals, by strangulation, which Stern has described, where there is always a stereotyped tendency to put on, or have on their person female clothing. There are numerous diseases in criminals and social deviants that we have not sufficiently studied.

Doctor Martin Hand: The term "epilepsy" is more or less a cliché that we use in referring to a type of apparent motor phenomenon. On the other hand, we also are aware of the fact that some disturbances in cerebral physiology can be manifested in other non-motor forms. The cases Doctor Revitch has discussed are chiefly behavioral disturbances. In electroshock therapy following treatment, we frequently encounter behavioral disturbances that cannot be easily distinguished from those that occur spontaneously in the syndrome that is called psychomotor epilepsy. Yet, occasionally, we see patients in treatment who are assumed to be mentally disturbed but who, in the midst of a rather continuous mental disturbance, manifest paroxysms of behavior which cannot be truly differentiated from the so-called psychomotor epilepsy.

If one does an EEG on such a patient, dysrhythmias will be found, sometimes with focal alterations in the temporal lobes.

My thought in the matter has been that some of these patients may represent a form of psychomotor epileptic status. Some of these patients, when treated with electric stimulation, will tend to normalize their behavior after a period of time. I have on record one patient who, after recovery, showed a normal tracing.

The fact that in most instances the electroencephalogram on psychotic patients shows little or nothing, should not preclude considering that some of them may be epileptics. The point that I wish to make is that even in motor epilepsy, there is a percentage of individuals who show no abnormalities in the electroencephalogram after various forms of stimulation.

If we were to weed out of the psychotics that we encounter, those patients with paroxysmal behavioral disturbances that seem to be occurring in the course of a more chronic type of mental disturbance, we might more frequently find patients that may be considered epileptic.

Doctor Eugene Revitch: As to the objection to calling these attacks psychomotor paroxysms, I must admit that I could not find another suitable word to describe them. I would like to stress that many of the patients with these attacks were originally diagnosed as cases of psychomotor epilepsy. To the second question of whether I used activation methods in the electroencephalograms, the answer is that unfortunately this was not possible, since the records were taken in various state laboratories and by various technicians. I believe that, as a general rule, a thorough history taking and clinical studies surpass electroencephalography in importance. For instance, the EEG of one of the patients showed slow bursts coupled with fast activity. Because of the record, she was diagnosed as a case of epilepsy. Yet, under hypnosis and sodium amytal, it was possible to determine the psychogenic nature of her fits.

As to whether I tried to control the seizures with anti-convulsive medication, the answer is that I actually took these patients off Dilantin, and obtained freedom from attacks by placing them in a different cottage or with different supervisors. A psychologist from New Jersey Prison Farms assisted me in a clinical follow-up of a prisoner with this type of seizure. This prisoner improved after withdrawal of Dilantin, just by placing him with a different supervisor.

To the question about suicide-strangulation among prison inmates, I must answer that I have not seen it so far. I would like to stress, however, the frequent occurrence of self-destructive tendencies which reminds me of two historical examples: Alexander the Great and Vincent VanGogh. Alexander the Great is described by Plutarch as a suspicious, paranoid personality. Not unlike the cases I had the opportunity to observe, he developed a fit of fury against his friend Clytus, whom he pierced with a spear. Immediately afterwards, he attempted to stab himself. The fit was connected with an outburst of paranoid ideation. VanGogh's fits were also outbursts of fury, stimulated by flashes of paranoid thinking. Cases of this sort cannot be diagnosed as psychomotor epilepsy and should be isolated as separate entities. The first two cases presented here did present with occasional epileptic-like attacks, yet most of these seizures were not epileptic but emotionally triggered release phenomena connected with physiological and psychological immaturity coupled with inability to inhibit strong impulses. The first case with a true temporal spike improved, not with medication, but with Reiter's electrostimulation.

REFERENCES

1. Schwade, E. D., & Geiger, S. G. (1956). *Dis Nerv Syst, 17*:307.
2. Gibbs, E. L., & Gibbs, F. D. (1951). *Neurology, 1*:136.
3. Courchet, J. L. (1954). *Le Bulletin Medical, 68*:197.
4. Gayral, al., Millet, G., Morone, P., & Turnin, G. (1956). *Ann Medico-Psychologiques, 114*:25.
5. Gowers, W. R. (1885). *Epilepsy and Other Chronic Convulsive Disorders.* New York: William Wood and Co., 1885.
6. Hill, D. (1944). *Proc R Soc Med, 37*:317.

Chapter 18

PAROXYSMAL MANIFESTATIONS OF NONEPILEPTIC ORIGIN: CATATHYMIC ATTACKS

The purpose of this paper is to report clinical observations of paroxysmal manifestations which present a problem of differential diagnosis with epileptic disorders. The Jacksonian concept of an epileptic attack as a clinical correlate of excessive neuronal discharge in the brain is now widely accepted. The scalp electroencephalograms (EEG's) are not always a reliable method of differential diagnosis, since the abnormal discharge may be recorded only with cortical or depth electrodes. Abnormal records were reported in normal,[1] in nonepileptics with psychogenic movement disorders,[2] in prison inmates,[3] and in psychiatric patients.[4] In a review of the literature on the subject, Ellingson[5] found that a significant rate of EEG abnormality is correlated with the group diagnosed as psychopaths and with aggressive behavior.

The diagnostic problem may be further complicated by the fact that the confines of epilepsy are not always clear. Gowers[6,7] even questioned the possibility of intermediate conditions and the possibility of hysteroid attacks being transformed into epilepsy. Notkin[8] points out, in his review, that previous authors (Steffens, 1900; Oppenheim, 1904) also believed in a spectrum of seizures extending from hysteria to epilepsy. This concept is now shared in France by Baruk,[9-11] Courchet,[12,13] and Gayral et al.[14] Guillain,[15] in a review of the literature on hysteria, pointed out the existence of paroxysmal phenomena which are neither epilepsy nor hysteria, precipitated by emotional and physiological factors and known in the French literature under the name of "crises

Source: Revitch, E. (1964). Paroxysmal manifestations of non-epileptic origin: Catathymic attacks. *Diseases of the Nervous System, 15*:662-670.

neuropathiques." Klotz et al.[18] and Borensteing[17] found hypocalcemia in their cases of "crises neuropathiques." Their cases had much in common with what Gowers[6] described under the name vaso-vagal attacks. These attacks are characterized by a sudden onset of epigastric oppression, pallor, prostration, changes in pulse rate, shivering, chattering of the teeth, coldness of the extremities, anxiety, feelings of unreality, respiratory distress, and parethesia of the extremities.

Most of the cases reported by the French authors present affective outbursts and complex automatisms with various degrees of alteration of consciousness. Bleuler[18] mentioned attacks of hypermotility, flushing and behavioral outbursts in schizophrenics and in prison inmates. These outbursts were followed by "sleepy exhaustion" and then by return to the original state.

In the American literature, only a few papers on the subject have appeared in recent years. McCullough and Ingram[19] described paroxysmal outbursts of panic and shaking and jerking of the extremities without loss of consciousness. These patients also had attacks of headache, temper tantrums and a family history of ictal emotions. Mehlman[20] described, in Puerto-Rican soldiers, sudden attacks of violence, agitation, self-mutilation, violent movements, posturing and confusion. Some of the cases reported in the paper seemed to me to be acutely disturbed schizophrenics. The problem of differential diagnosis between epilepsy and schizophrenia, in bizarre behavioral outbursts, was treated by Monroe[21] and Lorenz et al.[22] In Monroe's cases,[21] occasional rare grand mal and psychomotor seizures occurred in nine out of 20 patients with predominantly psychiatric symptomatology. Monroe states: "The mixture of symptoms suggests a diagnostic group intermediate between schizophrenia and epilepsy-disorders which are usually considered qualitatively different."

Chafetz and Schwab[23] presented a conceptual model of epileptic seizures consisting in a mixture of various degrees of psychological and neurological causes, with purely neurological causes on the one end of the spectrum and the purely psychological causes on the other end. They did not, however, mention intermediary seizures between purely psychological states and epilepsy. Williams[24] mentioned the difficulty of differential diagnosis between epileptic and non-epileptic phenomena when the epileptic discharge is at the highest levels of cerebral function. In these cases, there is a strong involvement of psychological functions. Seizures consisting of autonomic discharge and behavioral outbursts connected with 6 and 14 per second positive spikes were described by Gibbs and Gibbs[25] under the title "thalamic and hypothalamic epilepsy." Schwade and Geiger[26] question the epileptic nature of the thalamic and hypothalamic epilepsy, and they believe that the attacks are not epileptic but rhinencephalic release phenomena. The lack of inhibition by higher centers, and the release quality of the various outbursts, was mentioned by previous authors.[2,11,14]

Clinical Observations

Three types of episodic disturbances presenting, at times, an insoluble problem of differential diagnosis with epilepsy attracted my attention:

1. Catathymic attacks.
2. Short episodes of distractibility and inattention.
3. Episodes of perceptual alterations. This paper will deal only with catathymic attacks.

Catathymic Attacks

There is a great similarity between this group and cases reported previously under various names.[2,8,12,14,18,22] It is a heterogeneous group of a purely psychogenic and a mixture of psychogenic and organic etiology. I presented some of these cases under the name of psychomotor paroxysms of nonepileptic origin[27] at a meeting of the Eastern Psychiatric Research Association. Doctor Hans Strauss, in discussing the paper, strongly objected to the term psychomotor which he felt was specific for psychomotor epilepsy. In the light of this criticism, catathymic attacks, borrowed from French literature,[14] would seem to be more appropriate.

Originally, I was confronted with these cases at the New Jersey prison system and later at the New Jersey State Diagnostic Center, private practice and at Lyons V.A. Hospital. All of the cases were seen more than once and several were followed from three to 10 years. Psychiatric and neurological examinations and routine EEG's were performed on all the patients. Sleep tracings, interviews with intravenous sodium amytal, and in various stages of hypnosis, was performed only in selected cases. Only in the New Jersey Reformatory for Women was the total inmate population available for statistical studies, while elsewhere the cases were examined as they were encountered in the course of routine duties.

The episodes consist of outbursts of seemingly unprovoked rage with various degrees of alteration of consciousness, assaultiveness, destructiveness and self- destructiveness. Patients may cut themselves with sharp objects and, on one occasion, I observed a female patient cut her breasts with a piece of glass. These outbursts may be followed or preceded either by limpness and falling down or by disorganized, purposeless thrashing of the extremities. Bi-temporal, throbbing headache, tightness in the chest and a feeling of suffocation prior to the seizures was described by some patients. These outbursts seem to be so much out of context to the casual observer that the diagnosis of psychomotor epilepsy was made in many instances.

Prolonged observation, intimate knowledge of the institutional environment and of the patients, hypnotic sessions, and sodium amytal interviews, usually bring to the surface the emotional content and the precipitating causes of these episodes. The importance of lengthy observations was already mentioned by Lorenz et al.,[22] and the value of sodium amytal interviews in the diagnosis of bizarre seizures was mentioned by Collings.[28] The majority, but not all patients, presenting with these outbursts have personality traits marked by paranoid projections, suspiciousness and hostility. Courchet[13] also reports paranoid traits in his cases. In the study conducted at the New Jersey Reformatory for Women, 15 out of the 326 inmates presented with catathymic attacks. All of the 15 had paranoid personality traits, while only four out of 20 inmates selected at random, presented similar characteristics. The age of the inmates ranged from 16 to 75 years. The age distribution of the inmate population is reported in Table 18.1. The age distribution of the patients with catathymic attacks is reported in Table 18.2.

Table 18.1.
AGE DISTRIBUTION OF INMATE POPULATION

Age	Number of Inmates
16-22 years	101
20-35	157
Above 35 years	68

Table 18.2.
AGE DISTRIBUTION OF THE PATIENTS WITH CATATHYMIC ATTACKS

Age	Number of Patients
28 years	1
25 years	1
21 years	2
20 years	3
19 years	5
18 years	2
17 years	0
16 years	1
	Total = 15

Thus, the younger group was affected. An impression was gained that these outbursts have a tendency to disappear with age, maturation, and better motivation. An older inmate at the reformatory gave a history of behavioral outbursts diagnosed as epilepsy in her adolescence. She stated the following: "I was depressed. I wanted to be with my mother. Nothing mattered. I was upset. It was mostly nerves, but now I can control my temper." A young adult male in the Rahway Reformatory stopped similar attacks when reassigned to a sympathetic supervisor. A 19-year-old female inmate at the Reformatory for Women stopped her attacks with improved motivation in anticipation of positive parole board action.

Full scale IQ on the Wechsler-Bellevue Scale ranged from 63 to 115 with seven patients having IQ's over 90 and four over 80. Thus, only four patents could be considered mentally defective. Only four patients had EEG abnormalities consisting of (1) delta bursts and beta activity, (2) occipital slow dysrhythmia, (3) focal delta activity, and(4) sharp beta activity.

In the cases at the Reformatory for Women, the diagnosis of epilepsy was definitely eliminated in spite of abnormal EEGs in some. In other cases, an occasional automatism, suggestive of psychomotor epilepsy and rare grand mal seizures, were suspected in the history. In all the cases followed in the prison system, the episodes were of short duration lasting from one-half hour to a few hours, including the stage of mounting tension, the attack itself and the relaxation characterized by fatigue and somnolence. However, a series of cases with complex psychiatric symptomatology were observed among Veterans Administration patients whose attacks of rage were preceded by several days to a week of increasing suspiciousness, delusional elaborations, depression, and irritability.

CASE HISTORIES

Six representative cases from various sources of referral are chosen for illustration. The first three illustrate the group characterized by a relatively rapid evolution of the various phases of the outburst, while Cases 4 and 5 illustrate the more complex group with psychotic symptomatology and slow evolution. The attacks in Case 6 are connected with an anterior temporal spike and a temporal type of an aura, and thus are considered to be epileptic. The total personality organization is, however, closely related to Cases 4 and 5.

Case 1

A 17-year-old boy was admitted to the New Jersey State Diagnostic Center following several episodes of blind rage and destructiveness with what seemed to have been loss of awareness of the environment. During one episode, he fell down the stairs and sustained fracture of his hand. After admission to the local hospital, he was diagnosed as "traumatic psychomotor disorder," since two years prior to the incident he was in a car accident in which his mother had been killed, but he was not injured. Upon admission to the Diagnostic Center, he displayed aggressive behavior and he continued having episodes of violent rage triggered by insignificant incidents. Neurological examination and routine and sleep EEG's were normal. On the Wechsler-Bellevue test, he scored a full scale IQ of 94. The projective tests, according to the psychologist, revealed "affect always close to the surface in form of excitement", as well as fantasies of being overwhelmed and destroyed.

In psychiatric interviews, he spoke about "being pushed around by everybody", of being "walked over like dirt by everybody," and so forth. He said he had temper tantrums since the age of eight years but only recently developed the episodes he called "violent strokes." After provocation, he feels dizzy, nauseous and tense. Then he lies down and breathes heavily. After that, he has feelings like "getting hot inside my head, like the sun looking at you. After that, I don't remember." In a hypnotic state, he spoke about hatred toward the driver who caused the accident in which his mother lost her life, and he reenacted a dialogue with his mother when she did not meet his demands. He then began breathing heavily. This was followed by reenactment of a typical rage outburst.

Case 2

A 33-year-old male serving a sentence at Trenton State Prison for breaking and entering and larceny was referred for evaluation because of outbursts of rage which were thought to be of epileptic nature. The patient had a record of violence and fighting and he previously had served a sentence on a conviction for rape. He was discharged from several jobs because of explosive and violent behavior. On one occasion, he attacked his employer with a knife when the latter criticized his work. On another occasion, while working on the docks, he threw a hook at a fellow worker. In a fit of anger, he attempted to throw his wife out of a window, and another time, he attempted to choke her. Once, in a fit of anger, he struck a child on the street when a marble accidentally hit him. He felt that this was deliberate, but after the explosion of temper, he felt sorry and bought a hot dog for the child. During a previous imprisonment, he was hit on the head with a pipe in a fight.

Although there was no loss of consciousness or serious injury, he developed pulsating, bi-temporal headache, gradually invading the frontal region with a faint buzzing, gradually increasing in intensity. This was followed by an increase of general tension, sweating, and an urge to destroy, then an episode of violence without loss of consciousness. During one attack, he broke windows; on another occasion, he had an impulse to cut himself with a razor blade. He felt that the best way to handle these episodes was to be left alone. He claimed that he had a desire to kill and, when someone looked at him "the wrong way," "I want to choke the guy for nothing. When I hear the buzzing I think kill-kill." He said he trusted people as long as "they don't fool me" and, therefore, he avoids closeness to people. In interviews, his affect was warm and there was no loss of contact and no detachment. In the prison he gambled and made attempts to manipulate inmates and officers. On Wechsler-Bellevue test, he scored a full scale IQ of 79. On the

Rorschach, he gave responses such as blood, pus, poison . . . fighting and charging animals, and so forth. On routine EEG, a low voltage fast pattern was revealed. Repeated examinations could always prove a precipitating cause for his outbursts. He improved when he was assigned to a yard detail.

Case 3

This patient is now a 27-year-old married mother of a child, and has been free of outbursts of violence for about seven years. She was first admitted to the New Jersey State Diagnostic Center at the age of 13 for evaluation of sexual promiscuity. At the age of 15, she returned as an outpatient for evaluation of outbursts of uncontrollable rage followed by falling down on the ground and possible loss of consciousness. The attacks started at the age of 14 years, a few months after the death of her father. She, however, was known to have had less dramatic temper tantrums since the age of seven years. At the age of 17, she was committed to the reformatory for women and I had the opportunity to continue personal contacts until her 22nd year.

On the surface, the attacks seemed to be unprovoked, but in interviews with sodium amytal and under hypnosis, it was revealed that the attacks were preceded by frustrating experiences. In one interview, she said, "I keep everything inside. I do not trust my feelings. I seem happy but no one knows I am depressed." Headaches, crying spells and feelings of being hurt precede an outburst. The subjective experience of the attack was described: "I cannot breathe and I pass out. It seems that if I could cry, I would not have the seizure, but I do not cry." She reported an incident preceding an attack: "A day before the last spell two girls ran away. The whole lot of them were hollering and screaming and I was blamed. Mrs. H. (the supervisor) told me I was going to be removed from my cottage. My best girlfriend was in that cottage, so I started crying and hollering. I had a headache. The girls tried to calm me. Then I had a seizure." In a hypnotic state, she recollected her first attack at age 14: "I was in a camp. I had a terrible headache. I wanted to lie down and I started to cry. My legs felt as if they were not here. I could not breathe and I passed out." This attack was also precipitated by a feeling of being hurt and slighted which she described: "We put on an entertainment and I wanted to sing. I messed up the song and they all laughed. I was mad and I was hurt." On one occasion, after an altercation with a supervisor, she became enraged, started crying and attempted to cut her wrists. The attacks disappeared at the age of 19 years in anticipation of a favorable parole action.

She returned to the reformatory at the age of 22, after an assault on her boyfriend. She claimed she no longer had the outbursts described before. She became religious and remained compliant, cooperative, and free of attacks until now (age 27 years). I last examined her when she was 22 years old. She then told me the following in describing the outbursts: "I didn't care what happened to me. I felt no one loved me. It was a mad fit of temper. Heavy breathing made me pass out. I stopped it because I made up my mind." She claimed that she now felt at peace with herself, since she came to the realization that her mother liked her, while previously she believed that she was disliked by her.

The EEG's taken at the age of 15, 18, and 19 years showed a similar pattern of hypersynchronous delta bursts and runs of Beta activity. At the age of 22 years, only isolated theta waves were elicited in a routine record. She was originally treated with anticonvulsives by her family physician, yet the attacks have ceased in spite of the removal of medication.

Case 4

This patient was first examined and treated at the age of 32. The episodes start with moodiness, irritability, sullenness, withdrawal, depression and unfounded accusations of unfaithfulness, coldness, and rejection by his wife. The tension increases for about one week and ends with a feeling of "explosiveness in the stomach," immediately followed by an outburst of violent and destructive rage lasting about half an hour. Then, for a period of several days, there is depression and self-accusations. In the years following discharge from the hospital, suspicion of his wife's infidelity increased, and he complained that she did not satisfy him sexually while he reported a marked decrease in potency. The wife believed that he had no attacks when he could have his way. She always doubted his claim of amnesia for the violent phases of the episodes. Attacks stopped when his wife finally left him and he had full freedom of outside activities. At this time, seven years after our first contact, he told me: "I feel as if the pressure is off. I am doing now what I always wanted to do, such as horseback riding. I now do things I gave up when I was married." He also claimed that previously he was unable to talk back to people, but later he learned to talk back to superiors at work and this helped him to relax. Sometime after discharge from the V.A. Hospital, it was necessary to admit him to a sanitarium because of mounting tension which ended with an attack of violence in the admission office. Years later, he reported that an argument with his wife precipitated this episode. It is noteworthy that attacks started five months after his marriage. His EEG's were either normal or characterized by flat top 5 per second waves or burst-like activity in the left temporal leads.

Case 5

This patient was first examined and treated at the age of 31 and reexamined and followed for a period of one year, 10 years later. His outbursts started after a harrowing experience during the war when his ship was torpedoed and his friends killed. Right after the incident, he became irritable and intolerant of noise. Upon evacuation to the United States, he cried easily and he could not control his emotions. He frequently had an urge to scream and to smash things. The first attack of violence took place while he was on leave from the naval hospital. Earlier in the day, he received sedation because of mounting tension. In the hotel room, he suddenly became violent; he struck the wall with his fist, he pulled out his hair, and it took four people to restrain him. At the original examination, he claimed he had no recollection of the episode, but ten years later he said, "I remember a feeling of anger and tension. I felt I had to let it out like a steam kettle. Next thing, I started pounding the wall. I got exhausted from anger and I passed out."

Two years after discharge from the Navy, he reenlisted in the Air Force since he felt he could not make an adjustment to civilian life. After two years of service, he was given a medical discharge following another episode of violence triggered by the crash-landing of his plane. He described this experience s follows: "the plane crashed in landing. I was knocked down for a few seconds and when I came to, I was in the base hospital. The next thing, I blew my top and started to tear the hospital apart, knocking holes in the wall and throwing things around." The attacks of violence that occurred after the discharge from the air force started in a stereotyped pattern of mounting tension, irritability, headaches, depression, crying spells, suspiciousness and fleeting paranoid delusions, lasting days, sometimes weeks. This was followed by a short-lived, but intense attack of violence and ended with a feeling of guilt and suicidal thoughts lasting a few days. In addition to these attacks, there were also episodes of leaving home and wandering around the country, frequently getting into trouble with the police. He gave as a reason for suddenly leaving home, negative feelings evoked by his wife. Marital relations were stormy and pathological. He forces his wife to indulge in homosexual relations with other women or to entice men. During sexual relations, he wanted her to tell details about her previous sexual experiences. He himself, in childhood, had incestuous relations with his sister and, possibly, with his mother. On two occasions, he attacked a woman with a toy revolver. Yet, in hypnosis, he expressed great guilt over aggression. He became upset and emotional in revisualizing the shooting of a Japanese woman.

The EEG taken originally when he was 32 years old, showed hypersynchoronous bursts and negative sharp waves in the left mid-temporal region. Ten years later, several routine EEG's showed normal tracings consisting of 11-11½ per second alpha activity posteriorly, and sleep EEG's showed normal sleep patterns.

Case 6

This patient was first examined at the age of 32 for paroxysmal manifestations. He would suddenly become excited, fall on the floor, scream, thrash his arms and legs, and fight those who approached him. The attacks were ushered in by epigastric sensations and a peculiar surging upward from his legs. At the same time, or after these sensations, he experienced a vision of a halo surrounding a candle or a gun pinhole. Following this, he blacked out and had no recollection of the episode. The first attack occurred in combat in North Africa during World War II, and it was preceded by diffuse headache and tension. The patient was usually disheveled, suspicious, and subject to temper tantrums since childhood. According to his wife, he was impulsive, childish, and demanding. He was in several hospitals where he received diagnoses such as schizophrenia and psychopathic personality.

Routine EEG's were all normal with 9½-10 per second alpha activity dominating posteriorly. In light stages of sleep, however, a negative spike in the left anterior temporal region was found consistently, with phase reversal in other leads in monopolar recordings with the ears as a reference. Neurological examination and pneumoencephalogram were normal. I saw him again eight years later at the New Jersey State Diagnostic Center for evaluation because of an incestuous relationship with his daughter. He then revealed that he took no medication for almost eight years, since his discharge from the Veterans Hospital, and that his attacks ceased completely when his wife left him and he felt free. Only in jail, he again experienced epigastric sensations and a feeling of surge. The psychometric tests revealed a full scale IQ of 112 on Wechsler-Bellevue Scale, while the projective tests revealed hostility, distrust, defensiveness, sexual inadequacy, and resentment against females.

COMMENT

The cases reported here, under the title of catathymic attacks, belong to a heterogeneous group of conditions having in common episodes of behavior disturbances which pose a problem of differential diagnosis, etiology, and mechanism of the attacks.

Differential Diagnosis

Unless the attacks are preceded by an aura of motor manifestation, referable to a focus in the temporal lobe or to the structures in or around the sylvian fissure (and is connected with an anterior temporal spike,[29] diagnosis may be difficult or even impossible without careful neuropsychiatric follow-up. What has to be determined is whether the paroxysmal phenomena are due to a neuronal discharge or another cause.

The catathymic attacks seem to evolve in three stages: (a) mounting tension, (b) outburst, and (c) relief. In the catathymic attacks, a relationship with a precipitating event and with environmental influences is more intimate and obvious than in psychomotor epilepsy. Influence of environmental factors and emotional stimuli in psychomotor epilepsy was reviewed by Chessik and Bolin.[30] In catathymic attacks, the ability to control the episodes, with a change of motivation and surroundings can frequently be demonstrated. Throbbing headache during the stage of mounting tension, a feeling of tightness in the chest, feelings of suffocation, and hyperventilation in the initial stages of the episode, are common.

Several patients described epigastric sensations as churning or explosive, directly related to the general experience of tension. The epigastric aura in psychomotor epilepsy is, on the contrary, perceived as a surge and as alien to the total experience (Case 6). Cases 4, 5, 6 were initially reported as epileptics with psychiatric manifestations.[31] Extramural follow-up, after discharge from the hospital, led me to believe that only Case 6 could be diagnosed as psychomotor epilepsy. In Cases 4 and 5, the quality of intimate connection of the episodes with emotional stimuli, the perception of the episodes by the patients as attacks of anger, the perception of the experience as ego-syntonic rather than ego-alien, and failure to respond to anticonvulsives, forced me to change the diagnoses from epilepsy to a nonepileptic condition. These cases seem to be related to the episodic psychoses of Kleist (episodische "dammerzustande") cited by Strauss.[22] Kleist believed that these states were related to, but not identical with, epilepsy. According to Strauss,[22] it is not clear "how many of these episodic psychoses would be classified as truly epileptic today."

Etiology

In many cases, temper tantrums since childhood and disturbances of behavior are a common finding. A traumatic event frequently precedes the acute episodes. The following events preceded the attacks in cases used as illustrations: Case 1–death of mother, Case 2–slight head injury in a fight, Case 3–death of father, Case 4–marriage and marital discord, Case 5–combat experience and crash landing of his plane. In Cases 4 and 5, attacks were usually precipitated by marital strife caused by the patients' disturbance in the psychosexual area.

Mechanism of Attacks

While an epileptic seizure is a correlate of a cerebral discharge, catathymic attacks are emotional release phenomena connected with poor ability to control, to inhibit, and to redirect emotional impulses into constructive activity. Depending on the personality organization and the state of the central nervous system, the emotional release may be of such intensity that control is impossible and the outburst seems to be involuntary. In some cases, control is possible and patients improve with better attitudes and reorientation of goals. These patients may tell you, years later, that the outbursts were "a mad fit of temper" and that "heavy breathing made me pass out" (see Case 3). In a previous paper,[27] I divided the attacks into four etiological groups, placing in group 1, the purely physiological causes such as hypoglycemia, and in Group 4, the purely psychological causes, such as conversion reactions. The catathymic attacks occupy the transitional area of the spectrum.

Chessik and Bolin[30] ascribe to psychomotor seizures the function of maintaining internal homeostasis. I believe that epileptic seizures do not serve a function but are a result of a cerebral discharge. The discharge may be provoked by an emotional stimulus. Lennox[33] expressed this concept as follows: "As a gun may be fired by a very slight pressure of the trigger, convulsions may be set off by emotional disturbance." In catathymic attacks, the emotional outbursts do seem to serve the economic function of maintaining internal homeostasis. Abnormal EEG's, in some of the cases, indicate either immaturity or some defect in cerebral organization which makes it impossible to withstand hostile tensions without a discharge. In other cases, the personality organization is so loose and immature that tensions have to be discharged violently. This explains why, in cases observed among the female inmates of correctional institutions, the attacks had a tendency to disappear with age. Cases in which infrequent grand mal or possibly psychomotor seizures were observed can be explained. A high threshold epileptogenic focus may be fired on occasions by a strong emotional stimulus. The focus, in its turn, interferes with the ability of the brain to handle tensions and hence the occurrence of catathymic attacks.

SUMMARY

A heterogeneous group having in common episodes of behavioral disturbance was described under the name of catathymic attacks. Differential diagnosis with psychomotor seizures consists in intimate connection of these attacks with emotional triggers. Whereas epileptic phenomena are correlates of a cerebral discharge, catathymic attacks are considered to be emotional release phenomena. Their function is to maintain internal homeostasis in patients with an immature personality make-up or with a defective central nervous system organization.

These patients are unable to withstand an accumulation of hostile tension, yet they have the possibility of control with better motivations and with aging and maturation. Five illustrative cases were presented. Case 6 with psychomotor seizures was presented for contrast and comparison.

REFERENCES

1. Gibbs, F. A., Gibbs. E. L., & Lennox, W. G. (1943). Electroencephalographic classifications of epileptic patients and control subjects. *Arch Neurol Psychiat, 50*:111.
2. Kessler, M. M., Halle, L., Evans, M. W., & Shelton, W. R. (1952). Psychogenic motor phenomena in the presence of an abnormal electroencephalogram. *J Nerv Ment Dis, 116*:1.
3. Silverman, D. (1944). The electroencephalogram of criminals. *Arch Neurol Psychiat, 52*:38.
4. Kennard, M. (1953). The electroencephalogram in psychological disorders: A review. *Psychosom Medic, 15*:95.
5. Ellingson, R. J. (1954). The incidence of EEG abnormality among patients with mental disorders of nm organic origin: A critical review. *Am J Psychiat, 111*:263.
6. Gowers, W. R. (1907). *The Borderland of Epilepsy,* P. B. Blackiston, Son and Co. Philadelphia.
7. Growers, W. R. (1885). *Epilepsy and other chronic convulsive diseases.* New York: William Wood & Co.
8. Notkin, J. (1930). Affectepilepsy and hysteroepilepsy: A study of convulsive states in psychopaths. *J Nerv Ment Dis, 72:* 266.
9. Baruk, H. (1944). *Annales Medico-Psychologiques, 102*:275.
10. Baruk, H. (1933). *J Belge de Neurologie et de Psychiatrie, 33*:139.
11. Baruk, H. (1959). *Traite de Psychiatrie* Vol II Chapt. XI. Paris: Masson et Co. Editeurs.
12. Courchet, J. L. (1954). *Le Bulletin Medical, 68*:197.
13. Courchet, J. L. (1955). *Ann Medicao-Psychologiques, 113*:28.
14. Gayral, L., Millet, G., Moran, P., & Turnin, J. (1956). *Ann Medico-Psychologiques, 114*:25.
15. Guillain, G. (1941). *La Semaine des Hopitaux, 14*:1248.
16. Klotz, H. P., Borenstein, P., & Ribiere, G. (1949). *La Semaine de Hospitaux de Paris, 26*:625.
17. Borenstein, P. (1949). *La Semaine des Hopitaux de Paris, 26*:640.
18. Bleuler, E. (1952). *Dementia Praecox or the Group of Schizophrenias.* New York: International Universities Press.
19. McCullogh, W., & Ingram, W. Jr. (1956). *Dis Nerv Syst, 17*:279.
20. Mehlman, R. D. (1961). The Puerto Rican syndrome. *Am J Psychiat, 118*:328-332.

21. Monroe, R. R. (1959). Episodic behavioral disorders: Schizophrenia or epilepsy? *Archives of Gen Psychiat, 1*:205.
22. Lorenz, J. C., Levy, L., David, J. F., & Eng, M. (1962). *Comprehensive Psychiat, 3*:54.
23. Chafetz, M. E., & Schwab, R. S. (1959). Psychological factors involved in bizarre seizures: Report of four cases. *Psychosom Med, 21*:96.
24. Williams, D. (1956). The structure of emotions reflected in epileptic experiences. *Brain, 79*:29.
25. Gibbs, E. L., & Gibbs, F. A. (1951). Electroencephalographic evidence of thalamic and hypothalamic epilepsy. *Neurology, 1*:136.
26. Schwade, E. D., & Geiger, S. G. (1956). Abnormal EEG findings in severe behavior disorders. *Dis Nerv Syst, 17*:307.
27. Revitch, E. (1958). Psychomotor paroxysms of nonepileptic origin. *Dis Nerv Syst, 19*:562.
28. Collings, H. Jr. (1958). *Neurol Psychiat, 89*:408.
29. Gibbs, E. L., Gibbs, F. A., & Fuster, B. (1948). Peculiar temporal localization of sleep-induced seizure discharges of psychomotor type. *Arch Neurol Psychiat, 60*:331.
30. Chessik, R. D., & Bolin, R. R. (1962). Psychiatric study of patients with psychomotor seizures. *J Nerv Ment Dis, 134*:72.
31. Revitch, E. (1954). Epileptic manifestations resembling psychiatric disorders. *J Med Soc New Jersey, 51*:3.
32. Strauss, H. (1959). Epileptic disorders. In S. Arieti, *American handbook of psychiatry*, New York: Basic Books, Inc.
33. Lennox, W. G. (1944). Seizure states, in J. Hunt, *Personality and behavior disorders.* New York: Ronald Press.

Chapter 19

EPILEPTIC AND NONEPILEPTIC PAROXYSMS: A PROBLEM OF DIFFERENTIAL DIAGNOSIS

In connection with a legal action a few years ago, New Jersey physicians were dismayed by the discovery of a 1912 law which required the reporting of epileptic patients to boards of health. This precipitated a rush of reports not only of cases with seizures but also of patients with paroxysmal manifestations of nonepileptic origin. For this reason, a review of the concept and diagnosis of epilepsy and of nonepileptic paroxysm seems to be timely.

The Jacksonian concept of an epileptic seizure as being a clinical correlate of an excessive neuronal discharge is now widely accepted. The difference between an epileptic and nonepileptic paroxysm is simply the presence (or absence) of an excessive electrical discharge in the brain. Nonepileptic paroxysms are an expression of emotional release through motor activity or of perceptual and somatic concomitants of anxiety. In addition, there are attacks (chiefly of an organic nature or remotely connected with emotions) such ah hypoglycemia, narcolepsy (particularly attacks of cataplexy), migraine, and fainting spells that should be considered in the differential diagnosis.

Diagnostic Problems

Paroxysmality and altercations of consciousness are the cardinal symptoms of epilepsy. Unless the clinical picture is classical and clear-cut, this may be insufficient for a definitive diagnosis. There is an array

Source: Revitch, E. (1970). Epileptic and non-epileptic paroxysms: A problem of differential diagnosis. *Journal of the Medical Society of New Jersey*, *67*:635-638.

of bizarre psychogenic seizures resembling grand mal. Minor and psychic attacks may present a difficult and, at times, insoluble problem of differential diagnosis. Emotional precipitation of these attacks can be usually elicited with meticulous psychiatric investigation, but even this is not assurance that the seizures are non-epileptic. Many epileptic seizures may be emotionally precipitated.[1] There is a whole spectrum of bizarre epileptic seizures with various degrees of emotional and organic components.[2] The diagnostic difficulties in cases involving psychologic functions were stressed by Williams.[3]

Electroencephalography is an invaluable adjunct to out diagnostic armamen-tarium, but it is not always helpful and, at times, it may be confusing. The reasons for these failures is as follows: (a) an abnormal discharge may be recorded with depth electrodes only (essentially a neurosurgical or an experimental procedure), (b) routine records may be normal while activating procedures such as induced sleep, intravenous injection of metrazol, or photic stimulation may elicit a focal or generalized abnormality, (c) artifacts and technical errors may be misread as abnormal discharges, and (d) abnormal records in non-epileptics may be associated with nonepileptic motor or psychic paroxysms (4, 5, 6). Furthermore, the boundaries of epilepsy are not always clear. Thus, the 6 and 14 per second positive spikes described by Gibbs and Gibbs[7] as associated with behavioral and autonomic outbursts were thought to be diagnostic of what they named thalamic and hypothalamic epilepsy. Subsequently, it was found that this EEG pattern may be familial and may be seen in adolescents without the clinical picture described by Gibbs. Consequently, many doubts were expressed as to the epileptic nature of the entity. Henry[8] states that "the real clinical significance of this pattern, if there be any, is anything but clear." His experience suggests that "bursts of positive spiking might be regarded as a neurophysiologic handicap, the importance of which varies as function of the environment." Schwade and Geiger[9] also criticized the "epileptic" theory of this pattern and they felt that the attacks were due to rhinencephalic release phenomena, i.e., there were emotional outbursts due to poor physiologic control mechanisms.

Neurological examination, spinal fluid, and contrast studies rarely enlighten the practitioner, unless the seizures are due to a space occupying mass. In some psychoanalytic and psychologic circles, epilepsy is considered to be a specific entity with a specific personality make-up which can be elicited with projective tests. Lennox[1] and most epileptologists believe this to be untrue. Of all the diagnostic steps, a thorough history, with a scrupulous recording of the seizures, is the most important. Presence of an aura or of initial motor phenomena (such as adversive movements or Jacksonian march) related to a specific focus of discharge indicate, without fail, the epileptic origin of a seizure. The diagnosis of complex psychiatrically tinged seizures is impossible without a thorough knowledge of brain anatomy. This knowledge enables the clinician to deduce the initiation and spread of the discharge in the brain through observable clinical manifestations. Such an anatomo-clinical correlation, wherever it can be established, is the most certain diagnostic criterion. The following case may serve as illustration:

Case 1

A 32-year-old male had attacks of falling down, rolling on the floor, thrashing around, and fighting those who approached him. EEGs were normal. The attacks seemed to be of an emotional rather than epileptic nature. At a later date, a thorough anamnesis elicited epigastric sensations and visual hallucinations preceding the attack. This type of aura corresponds to a discharge starting in the sylvian fissure and spreading to the temporal area. In fact, an abnormal record (anterior temporal spike) was recorded in light sleep, but this followed the diagnosis established through clinical means.

Lennox,[1] in a discussion from the floor at one of the meetings, stressed the frequent diagnostic uncertainties and the necessity of prolonged observation in complex and bizarre seizures.

Nonepileptic Attacks

Cases of nonepileptic attacks and their diagnostic problems were recently reported by Liske and Foster[10] and Ferris.[11] These authors, however, did not make an attempt at classification and Ferris[11] just mentioned that the attacks "are of a type often called hysterical seizures." That not all of the nonepileptic seizures are "hysterical" was stressed by Guillain.[12] He described under the name of "crises neuropathiques" attacks which are neither hysterical nor epileptic. The authors, at the turn of the century, questioned the possibility of seizures, intermediate between epilepsy and hysteria, and they coined the phrase "hysteroepilepsy." The concept of intermediate seizures is still supported by some French authors.[5]

A mixture of epileptic and nonepileptic seizures in the same patient is a distinct possibility. In Monroe's 20 cases of nonepileptic attacks with predominantly psychiatric symptomatology, nine had occasional grand mal and psychomotor seizures.[13] In previous papers,[5,6] I divided the nonepileptic seizures into (a) catathymic attacks, (b) short episodes of distractibility and inattention, and (c) episodes of perceptual alterations. To this, one should add true hysterical attacks. Attacks are considered hysterical when they solve an inner conflict symbolically through motor activity. The *grande hysterie* of Charcot is a typical example. In these cases, the seizures may be prolonged and manifested by bizarre motility or by rigid postures, usually opisthotonos. The following case is representative:

Case 2

A 15-year-old boy had attacks of opisthotonos lasting 45 to 60 minutes. Prior to a seizure, he rushed to the school nurse, but never could reach to her office in time because of loss of control of his legs. Spells were preceded by sharp pain the chest. During the spell, breathing was noisy and rapid; or at times, he seemed to hold his breath and choke. He usually grunted and groaned and after the spell he staggered around the office for several minutes. His physician felt he needed immediate hospitalization to prevent "status epilepticus." In the course of therapy, it was discovered that the seizures were preceded by arguments with his mother. The patient was a strange, suspicious, and secretive boy. He had a particular attraction for reptiles and, on one occasion, he brought a valise with snakes to my office and let the snakes crawl on my desk. His seizures stopped later in life when he left home.

Catathymic attacks are referred to in the French literature.[5] They consist of behavioral outbursts considered neither hysterical nor epileptic. In most cases, the attacks present a diffuse uncontrolled and undirected expression of underlying rage. In many instances the attacks are preceded by a traumatic event. Emotional instability and outbursts of anger with assaultiveness and destructiveness are a common finding. A typical example, are cases of delinquent girls tearing off the radiator, cutting the breast with a piece of glass, or thrashing on the floor. I had the opportunity to examine such cases in correctional institutions. When the attacks seem to be unprovoked and patients allege amnesia following recovery, the differential diagnosis with psychomotor epilepsy is an obvious problem. Careful interview, particularly under the influence of intravenously injected sodium Amytal or in superficial stages of hypnosis, usually brings forth the emotional stimuli precipitating the attack. These attacks improve with maturation and with motivation. The following case is illustrative:

Case 3

A young adult male prisoner serving a sentence for breaking and entering had frequent attacks of violence preceded by pulsating bitemporal headache. This was followed by buzzing in the ears, sweating, and a feeling he had to destroy everything in his path. The attacks occurred mostly in crowds or when he felt trapped or enclosed. He had a history of emotional instability, inner tension, frequent outbursts of anger and homicidal impulses. He said, "I always wanted to kill. When I go down in the yard and somebody looks at me, I want to choke him." The Rorschach protocol reported aggressiveness and violence. His attacks were blind rages with poor recollection of the incidents. He improved with tranquilization and psychotherapeutic interviews. EEG was normal.

Short episodes of inattention may pose a differential diagnosis with petit mal and temporal lobe epilepsies. I found these phenomena mostly in children with distractibility, inattentiveness, and introversion.[6] One of these children, when first seen at the age of 10, was diagnosed elsewhere as a case of petit mal. His EEG, however, never showed the typical petit mal pattern, the attacks lasted 10 or more minutes, particularly when he was bored in school, and they finally stopped in late adolescence.

Short episodes of perceptual alterations are not uncommon in anxious and depressed individuals. The most commonly encountered manifestations are episodic feelings of unreality and derealization. The patient may feel unreal, distant, or in a fog. Others may present visual or kinesthetic illusions, particularly in states of reduced vigilance. Any stimulus arousing vigilance abolishes the sensation. The experience consists of attacks of macropsia, autoscopy, and changes of body size. The most common kinesthetic illusion I had the opportunity to observe was a feeling of acceleration of body functions and of the passing time. All of these phenomena may be seizure manifestations in temporal lobe epilepsies, part of the migraine syndrome, or they may be seen in psychiatric conditions.

Case 4

A 15-year-old boy had attacks of "strangeness and unreality" lasting 15 to 20 minutes. They were precipitated by rapid changes in the environment or through concentration. The boy was sensitive, introverted, anxious, and phobic. EEG was normal.

Cases 5 and 6

A sensitive, introverted 11-year-old girl and an albino 13-year-old boy had attacks so similar in appearance that both are reported together. Both, when reading or alone in a quiet room, experienced a feeling of extreme acceleration of their movements, body functions, and the passage of time. This could be interrupted through turning on the radio, joining the family in another room, or through stimulating activity. The episodes were accompanied by anxiety and both children were relieved with reassurance.

COMMENT

The area of differential diagnosis between epilepsy and nonepileptic paroxysms belies the spreading notion that psychiatry and neurology should be absolutely separated, and that the practice of psychiatry should follow a sociologic rather than medical model. It also confirms the value of the clinical approach and of neuropsychiatric rather than purely psychiatric or purely neurological perspective. Cushing[14] expressed the importance of clinical orientation in the following words: "We have instruments of precision in increasing numbers, with which we and our hospital assistants, at untold expense, make tests and take observations. The vast majority of these are but supplementary to, and as nothing compared with, the careful study of the patient by a keen observer using his eyes and ears and fingers and a few simple aids." In many instances of bizarre seizures, only cumulative evidence from a prolonged clinical follow-up leads to a final diagnostic formulation. Case 1 is an example of such an eventuality. Postictal sleepiness, headaches, and seizures occurring at night, particularly in the early hours of the morning upon awakening, are some other clues favoring an epileptic diagnosis. The complex seizures are not always easy to diagnose and, therefore, it is suggested that unqualified, precipitous reporting of patients with paroxysmal symptomatology is unwarranted.

SUMMARY

Epilepsy was defined in Jacksonian terms as a clinical manifestation of excessive neuronal discharge. The nonepileptic paroxysms may present pure emotional discharges or conditions such as cataplectic attacks of narcolepsy, manifestations of hypoglycemia, or various types of fainting spells due to emotional, vascular, or cardiac causes. The importance of clinical orientation and of the neuropsychiatric, rather than purely psychiatric or purely neurologic perspective, for successful diagnosis of ambiguous cases was stressed. It was suggested not to report patients as epileptics just because of paroxysmal nature of their condition.

REFERENCES

1. Lennox, W. G. (1944). Seizure states in Hunt's *Personality and the behavior disorders.* New York: Ronald Press.
2. Chafetz, M. E., & Schwab, R. S. (1959). Psychological factors involved in bizarre seizures: Report of four cases. *Psychosomatic Medicine, 21*:96.
3. Williams, D. (1956). The structure of emotions reflected in epileptic experiences. *Brain, 79*:29.
4. Kessler, M., Halle, L., Evans, M. W., & Shelton, W. R.(1952). *Journal of Nervous and Mental Diseases, 116*:1.
5. Revitch, E. (1964). Paroxysmal manifestations of nm-epileptic origin. *Diseases of the Nervous System, 25*:662.
6. Revitch, E. (1966). Epileptic manifestations resembling psychiatric disorders. *Diseases of the Nervous System, 27*:789.
7. Gibbs, E. L., & Gibbs, F. A. (1951). Electroencephalographic evidence of thalamic and hypothalamic epilepsy. *Neurology, 1*:36.
8. Henry, C. (1963). Positive spike discharges in the EEG and behavior abnormality, in Glaser's *EEG and behavior.* New York: Basic Books.
9. Schwade, E. G. & Geiger, S. G. (1956). Abnormal electroencephalographic findings in severe behavior disorders. *Diseases of the Nervous System, 17*:307.
10. Liske, E. & Foster, F. M. (1964). *Neurology, 14*:41.
11. Ferris, G. S. (1959). *Southern Medical Journal, 52*:1557.
12. Gullain, G. (1941). *La Semaine des Hôpitaux, 14*:1248.
13. Monroe, R. R. (1959). Episodic behavior disorders: Schizophrenia or epilepsy. *AMA Archives of General Psychiatry, 1*:205.
14. Cushing, H. (1933). *JAMA, 100*:1567, 20.

Chapter 20

SOCIAL ASPECTS OF EPILEPSY

Treatment of epilepsy is made up of two components: medical and psychologic social care. Therapy of epilepsy does not stop with anticonvulsive medication. It must be supplemented by psychologic therapy of the patient and by combating the prejudices of the public against epilepsy. That public attitudes toward this condition greatly interfere with social adjustment of epileptics is obvious to anyone who takes the trouble to become acquainted with the life history of epileptics. A survey of the attitudes of 2,696 adults[1] revealed that 92 percent of individuals read or heard about epilepsy; 24 percent would object to having their children associate with epileptics; and 25 percent felt that epileptics should not be employed in jobs like other people. The statistics also indicate that the higher the educational standard of the individual, the less hostile is his or her attitude toward the epileptic. In spite of a more favorable attitude evidenced by college graduates, a survey of 1,331 colleges[2] revealed that 21 percent of them admit epileptics conditionally and 14 percent do not admit them at all. The smaller the school the greater the reluctance to provide for epileptics. The eastern colleges are less willing to admit epileptics than are the colleges of the mountain and Pacific states. The survey also estimated that there are approximately 500 epileptic students in a college population of 1,000,000. However, assuming that one out of 200 citizens are epileptics, the number of epileptic students should be about 5,000.

Two-thirds of epileptics have normal mentality. A survey of 300 private patients by Collins and Lennox[3] shows that the average IQ (Wechsler-Bellevue test) was 112, and that a third of these patients had

---

Source: Revitch, E. (1951). Social aspects of epilepsy. *Journal of the Medical Society of New Jersey*, *48*:100-102.

an IQ of 120 and above. This suggests that most epileptics could be successful in college and perform various duties which are now denied them. To be sure, patients subject to convulsive seizures, or to lapses of consciousness (as in petit mal epilepsy), should not be permitted to drive a car or to occupy positions which would jeopardize their safety or the safety of others. They should be barred from such jobs as bus drivers, locomotive engineers, painters, brick-layers, pilots, and so forth. Unfortunately, one seizure–even in a "safe" occupation (such as a salesman in a store)–may mean loss of a job. The life of an epileptic child is particularly miserable. Some schools will not permit him or her to continue. Parents of an epileptic child, and epileptic adults themselves, may have a feeling of shame connected with their condition. This sense of shame, social ostracism, and danger of loss of a job, are responsible for the tendency of parents of epileptic children, and of adult epileptics, to keep the condition secret.

In a child, "fits" may be responsible for undue anxiety and overprotective attitudes on the part of the parents. Thus, the child is not permitted to participate in the normal activities of his age and is isolated from the companionship of normal children. During adolescence and the premarital period, epilepsy may interfere with courtship, marriage, and normal socialization of the young man or young woman, even if the seizures are very infrequent. Lennox[2] cites the case of a female student discovered by the college physician to have been taking Dilantin. She had been without a seizure for three years. In spite of that, she was forced to leave the college dormitory.

One of my patients at the Lyons New Jersey Veterans Hospital had a seizure in the lobby of a Y.M.C.A., where he was living. He was ordered to give up his room. Another veteran patient, a father of five children, with well controlled seizures with anticonvulsive mediation, obtained work as a counter-man at an ice cream parlor while he was on trial visit from the hospital. He lost the job as soon as the proprietor found out about his seizures. Those who have had skilled employment prior to the onset of illness are in a particularly deplorable situation because their unjust loss of their occupation may mean a considerable lowering of their family's standard of living. In my experience, only very few of these unfortunates were able to find other occupations and to readjust themselves to the new conditions. One automobile mechanic became a tailor, and a dental student with frequent petit mal attacks thought of changing from dentistry to law. Unfortunately, I have had no opportunity to follow these patients for any length of time after their discharge from the hospital.

The unfavorable attitudes toward epileptics is amply reflected in the literature. Lennox[4] in stressing the importance of social care of epileptics emphasizes, however, the obstacles such as prohibition of marriage of epileptics (in many states), discrimination by employers, and denial of education, particularly of higher education. Yet, 75 percent of epileptics can lead a normal life. Margaret Lennox[5] recently reported on a group of 22 employed epileptics: 15 of the 22 made an "adequate to good" work adjustment. Fourteen of the 22 made an "adequate to good" social adjustment. She finds that patients who are *not* secretive about their illness make better adjustments than those who deny it. Patients able to accept their illness have more self-confidence and self-respect than those who feel that they should keep it a secret. The Social Service department of Skillman Village in New Jersey, made an attempt to place epileptics on jobs. Here is what their case worker reported:[6] "Careful planning and effort were nullified when one of the men sent to apply for work had a seizure in the office of the personnel manager"; and "public employment agencies have shown a sincere interest in placing epileptic individuals but since they have been unable to place all applicants who do *not* have physical handicaps, they have found it almost impossible to place those who have a history of epilepsy"; and "continuing efforts have been made to interest farmers in accepting for employment men who are ready to go out on an extended visit, but no placements have been made for several years."

Administration of anticonvulsive medication is only one side of the treatment of epilepsy. Too many physicians limit themselves to prescribing anticonvulsive drugs without informing the patients about their illness and without any attempt to help them solve their emotional and social problems. This type of treatment is entirely inadequate. At the Lyons New Jersey Veterans Administration Hospital, there are "information meetings" with groups of nonpsychotic newly admitted epileptics. It is surprising how much anxiety is dispelled, and how much self-confidence and clearer perspective are gained, by that method. It is well-known to students of psychosomatics that emotion may precipitate fits. Contrariwise, a feeling of self-confidence and happiness will be very helpful in preventing seizures. Much of the frustrating experience of epileptics is due to public ignorance and family attitudes. An educational campaign is, therefore necessary. Is epilepsy a great enough problem for expenditures and efforts connected with attacking public prejudice? It is believed that there are about 600,000 epileptics in the United States and that about 50,000 veterans of both World Wars suffer from seizures. It is estimated[7] that in New Jersey alone there are about 20,000 epileptics. Only 10 percent of the epileptics are hospitalized. The rest are treated by private practitioners or in clinics. Hospitalized epileptics are less of a social problem than are outpatients because they constitute the bulk of the mentally deteriorated, or of those whose seizures occur at too frequent intervals for normal social or work adjustment.

What has been done for the solution of the problem involved in the social aspect of antiepileptic therapy? On the national scale, there were two lay societies, "The American Epilepsy League" and "The National Association to Control Epilepsy" which recently merged to form a unified organization now called "The National Epilepsy League."[8] Special efforts will be made by this league to establish epilepsy clinics, to draft a law that would provide for compensation to an epileptic injured at work, and to help children requiring special assistance in education. The National Epilepsy League, as well as its two parent societies, have published many pamphlets for the use of laymen interested in the subject. The physicians interested in epilepsy are organized in the "American League Against Epilepsy"[9] which is a branch of the "International League Against Epilepsy." The Medical Society of New Jersey and the State Department of Institutions and Agencies have recently developed a medico-social program for attacking the problem.[7] This program begins with the establishment of an advisory council, and a medical advisory committee, whose task will be to coordinate all private and public resources and to organize demonstration clinics for instruction and consultation services.

CONCLUSION

In spite of much progress in understanding the psychologic basis of epilepsy, and in developing of new anticonvulsive drugs, the care and treatment of epileptics will be incomplete without additional guidance of the patient, without dispelling his or her anxiety by providing an understanding of the illness, by fostering his feeling of self-esteem, and by changing public attitudes. This cannot be done by the private practitioner alone. Physicians, particularly neuro-psychiatrists, and also psychiatric social workers, will have to campaign through the press, radio, and lectures to the public, and through various medical societies. Their mission will be to acquaint the medical practitioner with some of the problems of epilepsy which otherwise may escape their interest or attention. The advisory council, as planned in the state of New Jersey, is a step toward the solution of the social therapy of epilepsy.

REFERENCES

1. Caveness, W. (1949). A survey of publications toward epilepsy. *Epilepsia, 4*:19.
2. Potter, G., McBride, M., & Lennox, W. (1949). *Proceedings of the national association to control epilepsy.* Baltimore, MD: Williams and Wilkins.
3. Collins, A. L., & Lennox, W. G. (1949) *Proceedings of the national association to control epilepsy.* Baltimore: Williams and Wilkins.
4. Lennox, W. G. (1947). Social therapy of epilepsy. *Canadian Medical Association Journal, 56*:638.
5. Lennox, M. A., & Mohr, J. (1950). Social work adjustment in patients with epilepsy. *American Journal of Psychiatry, 107*:257.
6. DeCamp, A. C. (1950). *The Welfare Reporter.* Published by the New Jersey Department of Institutions and Agencies, 4, 8, 9.
7. Unknown: (1950). A State Epilepsy Program. *Journal of The Medical Society of New Jersey, 47*:346. Also see the *Welfare Reporter* (1950). (N. J. Department of Institutions and Agencies) 5, 7, 8.

NAME INDEX

SUBJECT INDEX

Page numbers followed by t indicate tables.

N

T